DOCTOR HURDLE'S PROGRAM TO RETAIN YOUTHFULNESS

By the Same Author

*Low Blood Sugar: A Doctor's Guide to Its
Effective Control*

DOCTOR HURDLE'S PROGRAM TO RETAIN YOUTHFULNESS

J. Frank Hurdle, M.D.

Parker Publishing Company, Inc.
West Nyack, N. Y.

For Sheldon, Louise and Harriet

Printed in the United States of America
ISBN-0-13-216333-0
B & P

What This Book Can Do for You

Even before the days of Ponce De Leone who sought the Fountain of Youth, men have yearned to know the secrets of youth. Yet, these secrets have been right under the very noses of those who searched the world over in vain for their "Fountains of Youth." I intend to prove it to you in this book.

How would you like to look, feel, and stay younger, starting today? This book will show you just how to do so and with surprisingly little effort and with no gimmicks to buy or magic elixirs to gulp down.

I will demonstrate to you how you can begin to add fresh new days to your week. You will learn how to stretch these added weeks of new living into months then into years of revitalized youthful energy!

You can look in a mirror right now and tell if something should be done about your aging physique and rickety mind. Truthfully now, what do you see? A head of gray thinning hair set atop a prematurely wrinkled head with sagging jowls and several chins? Missing teeth? Caved-in chest with flabby muscles hanging everywhere about — muscles that have wilted with the years? Or perhaps an ever-expanding waistline with an apron of fat hanging over your groins? Maybe you don't look so badly, but how young do you feel? Brain dusty with those cobwebs covering what should be a vigorous, forceful creative mind? What about all those ideas and plans you've been going to put into action all this while — when did you last carry one of these plans out? Last month? A year ago? Five years?

Wouldn't you really like to regain some of that lost zip and spring in your step? That's what this book is all about. You'll soon learn how easy it really is and how good it makes you feel to stand straight and lithe once again — not only look like you put back some of those lost years, but really feel inside like you've completely reworked that carcass and that mind to the point where you are, literally, a newer, younger, person! This you can commence today — no further delays — no excuses using the same old worn out rationalizations — you can begin to be a younger individual *now*.

You know, all the much sought-after elixirs and Fountains of Youth aren't deeply hidden in some remote mountain cave on some even more remote and uncharted island. All the elixirs and potions you need for this remarkable transformation are right in your body at this very minute! You don't have to go on safari to find them. They're right there for the asking, if you will take the short time involved to learn what they are, how to reawaken them and keep them humming like a well-programmed computer for lasting and permanent youth!

In this book, you'll learn the secrets of your body's metabolism and how to prevent its aging you unnecessarily when you allow it to get out of whack. You'll learn how to master the art of physical conditioning and how this works as its own revitalizing super-charger to pump youthful energy to every cell in your body.

You'll learn how to keep a young creative mind, and how to tap your mind's vast resources of vibrant power. You'll also learn how to gain control of your body's inner cycles and electric potentials to keep your organism soaring at top efficiency and performance.

It seems that medical science comes up everyday with newer and more complex diseases that plague the human condition. In this book, I'll break down these diseases in simplified form and show you how to come through most diseases with flying colors, and, more importantly, how you can prevent nearly all the so-called crippling diseases before they ever get started!

Many people seem dismayed by the fact that they've let themselves "go too far already" to gain much help by mastering such knowledge. Don't believe it! This book is designed for all ages, 6 through 86, to help you regain and retain your youthful birthright.

I talked to a man of 40 not long ago who was completely resigned to looking, feeling and acting like he was 65. He is typical of hundreds I've seen. He was full of all sorts of fantasies about what happens to a person when he reaches 40 — if you listen to enough talk, of course, you begin to believe what others say even though they don't know what they're talking about. This gentleman was intelligent, held down an excellent job, had good physical potential, but a shameful-looking carriage. He was far from realizing youthful vigor, however. He was rapidly losing a head of graying brittle hair; he had three chins and wrinkles criss-crossing his wrinkles. He was soft, flabby and his eating and drinking habits were atrocious. He was, in fact, more sixty-fiveish than his forty years. On top of all this, he had recently been plunged neck-deep into the so-called generation gap with regard to his teen-aged children. This was the straw that broke his prematurely aging back.

When he began his trip back — began to grow healthy hair, began to get rid of his flabby exterior and replace it with solidly toned muscles, began to stir up his metabolic machinery to fine pitch — even the generation gap disappeared! He found out how to get on the same level with his children and speak as well as understand their language, fears, concerns and hopes. Both he and his family took a *younger* view and literally became *younger* for their efforts. Now both the children and the parents have great respect rather than hopeless contempt for one another.

All this and more can happen to you. Start bridging that generation gap of yours today by reading and applying the self-help in this book and gain the more youthful life you have been missing.

J. Frank Hurdle, M.D.

Contents

Step One: Your Body and How to
Restore Its Youth   (18)

*Your hide • Your frame • Your
"Innards"*

Fifteen Years Younger After Reverse
Aging   (20)

Step Two: Your Mind and How to
Keep It Youthfully Primed   (21)

Mind Power Restores Youth   (22)

Step Three: Mastering Your Youth
Cycles   (23)

Youth Cycles Pay Dividends for This
Man   (23)

Step Four: A Clean Bill of Health
for Vigorous Youth   (24)

A Double Indemnity in Health   (24)

Young Nerves and Organs Need
Energy   (26)

Involutional Melancholia
Reversed   (28)

The Road Back   (29)

**How to Take Four Big Steps Toward Looking,
Feeling and Remaining Younger (Continued)**

How to Build a Youthful Digestive and Elimination System in Your Body (Continued)

9. **Secrets of an Effective Breathing Method to Promote Youthfulness** **119**

10. **How to Keep Youthful Lustre in Your Skin, Hair, and Teeth** **135**

1

How to Take Four Big Steps Toward Looking, Feeling, and Remaining Younger

Of course you want to look and feel younger. Who wouldn't? Don't feel it's hopeless, and don't be discouraged by what you see in the mirror or because you got out of bed this morning only with the greatest effort. I want you to begin *today* to learn the easy way to youthful zip and bountiful energy. We'll begin by going over the four keystones of success in regaining youth and a brand new life of rippling strength, razor sharp thinking, cycle control and flawless health.

I'll show you how some people I know mastered these keystones and how easy it is for you to do exactly the same thing for yourself. You'll discover how to roll back the aging clock five, ten, even fifteen or more years! You'll find out how to utilize these four simple principles to reverse your aging pattern, stop falling hair, smooth out those wrinkles and restore a sparkle of youth to your eyes. What's more, you'll *feel* the difference. It won't be like merely having a face-lifting job or dying your hair — you'll *know* you are younger because *you will be younger*!

I'll discuss the correction of failing physique and the onset of disease with its flagging pep and drive. You'll find out how to regain that lost drive again only with double or triple its former intensity! I'll also tell you about people who rediscovered their minds — people who were slipping into senility, victims of their own ruts who failed to tap their own most precious natural resource — their minds. You'll find out how you can duplicate this feat with the result that years will literally tumble from you, and all your dried-up reservoirs will once again bubble over with youth reserves!

STEP ONE: YOUR BODY AND HOW TO
RESTORE ITS YOUTH

I'll wager it's been a long time since you've thought much about that carcass you travel around in every day except when it goes out of whack. Your body is the most amazing piece of machinery in the world. Take care of it, and the world can belong to you; abuse it, and bad news results. Of all the troubles confronting Americans today, their abuse of the human organism must head the list. And you might be surprised to find how much worn out bodies have to do with all the world's other problems!

Your Hide

Take your body's covering: hair, skin and connective tissue. Even if you might be fortunate enough to have youthful organs, if any of these three tissues becomes defective, you cannot help looking and feeling old.

To keep its natural lustre and smooth healthy appearance, your skin must be conditioned. It is a most amazing tissue and too often taken for granted until something comes along that causes it to malfunction. At this point, one regrets his neglect.

To remain young, *skin must retain its elasticity.* It's a lack of elasticity that causes skin to wrinkle, blemish and turn leathery. You've all seen people who aren't chronologically old with skin that looks and feels like the bark on a tree, or that appears thin and shiny. This can be avoided as we'll see later on in another section of this book. Since hair grows from skin, youthful looking hair depends on how you treat your skin.

Connective tissue is the layer of "stuff" separating skin from muscles. It is primarily of two classes — fat and fibrous tissue. I don't have to tell you how excessive deposits of fat age your organism. You can look at yourself and tell to what extent you've allowed the aging fat infiltration process to sneak up on you. Are there rolls of fat hanging down the front of your abdomen? When you extend your arm, does a blob of fat hang down, quivering like jelly from the underside of your upper arm? Without support, are your breasts drooping down toward your waistline? Buttocks vibrate when you walk from all the fat on them? You need to do some work! *Excess fat beneath your skin causes premature aging and, in turn, ages your skin as well.* I'll talk more in Chapters II and III on a vital youth-restoring method of keeping your body's fat within it's normal limit. You can add youthful years to your body by simply controlling its fat content!

Your Frame

Without a solid foundation and strong resilient support, a building crumbles to the ground. When its supports begin to sag, it's said to be aging. How true it is with your body! The main support and the foundation of its structure is bone and muscle and *the key to a youthful bony superstructure is in nutrition and conditioning.*

How could youth prevail without lithe trim muscles? It couldn't. You can regain years of youthful get up and go *by getting the tone back into those soft muscles!* This is done by conditioning — and it needn't occupy more than twenty or thirty minutes of your time each day with the week-end off! You will learn how this is done in section III.

Your "Innards"

Your body's vital organs — why has Nature in her wisdom seen fit to protect them all with either hard bone or the body's largest and thickest muscles? Because they perform the fantastic miracle of keeping you alive! Neglect them and the aging process sets in.

One of the most appalling parts of practicing medicine is to see a young person come dragging into the office looking and feeling twenty or twenty-five years older than his actual age. He has slipped into this rut through neglecting his vital insides. He has let his arteries and veins deteriorate, his nerves buckle, his gut winds itself up into knots, his heart weakens and his lungs collapse. He is an aged wreck!

But it isn't too late, even for this miserable soul — and there are hundreds of thousands of such people just like him who could be young again if they'd just take the time to revitalize their innards. This is done by desludging arteries and veins, injecting energy into nerves, turning a tight intestinal system into a smoothly humming nutritional dynamo and by pumping verve back into tired heart and lungs. I'll take each of these subjects up separately and show you how to get your aging innards young again.

FIFTEEN YEARS YOUNGER AFTER
REVERSE AGING

One of the most dramatic changes I've ever seen come over a person is the amazing case of Marge. This extremely sorry looking sight of a woman came into my office one day barely able to drag herself through the door. She was fifty years old and could easily have passed for seventy. She was about five feet three inches tall and weighed 203 pounds! She had dull straggly hair growing unkempt from a scaly dry scalp. She looked like the proverbial "wrath of God," with dark circles about her lusterless eyes. Sagging jowls pulled her mouth down into a constant scowl, and the rings of fat around her neck completely obliterated her Adam's Apple.

She really didn't walk, she waddled, and when she finally enveloped a chair in the waiting room, she was puffing like a locomotive. As she began to reel off her history and complaints, it became apparent that she was an example of what I call a "gold star museum piece." She had symptoms and disease in every system of her body and was currently on twelve different drugs for her ills! Her reason for coming in at the time, she said, was because she needed stronger pain medicine for the arthritis in her knees, hips and back.

I must confess I really hit the ceiling. I proceeded to "chew her up" one side and down the other. I lectured, scolded, even threatened her with the dire consequences of her present physical shape. I ended up with a flat refusal to prescribe stronger medicines. She'd heard some of this before, I feel certain, since she took the verbal chastising without blinking an eye. When she left, looking more like a floating haystack than human, I didn't think I'd ever see her again. About a week later she called and asked if I thought I could help. She said she'd decided she would do anything at all if she could be made to feel better again. I told her I couldn't make any promises, but if she was serious about "doing anything," I'd try my best.

In the hospital, tests and X-rays showed just about what I expected: abnormal loss of calcium from her bones, high fat levels in her blood, early diabetes from a failing pancreas gland, high blood pressure, failing heart and varicose veins in both legs. Truly, a sad looking body — an aged derelict of the worst kind.

First, to dispel her steadfast idea that she was "one of those people who just couldn't lose weight," I hospitalized her, severely restricted her diet and absolutely forbade visitors bearing parcels that could possibly contain food. After three weeks, Marge lost twenty-three pounds! The physiotherapy department started Marge on exercises, including hydrotherapy where she could start using muscles while submerged in water, thereby reducing effort and strain.

Marge was amazed how much she could do after only a week passed. After two weeks, the fat and sugar levels in her blood stream returned to near normal levels. Her blood pressure responded to weight loss well enough that she no longer needed drugs to control it. Her entire outlook changed so dramatically, and she was so successful with her weight reduction and conditioning routines at home that when I saw her in the office just under a year later, I couldn't believe my eyes. She had lost a total of seventy-five pounds, had literally cured herself of diabetes and hypertension and had gone to the beauty shop where her hair was done up such that it changed her entire appearance. Following a simple vein stripping in both legs, she hasn't had a sick day, and now heads a large group of "weights anonymous" for overweight women in her city. She does not look a day over thirty-five at the present time!

Marge's case is an exceptional one, but demonstrates an important point: *You have within you the potential to roll back years if you will take the time to do so!*

STEP TWO: YOUR MIND AND HOW TO KEEP IT YOUTHFULLY PRIMED

I've said it before and it's worth repeating: this country's most important and valuable natural resource is the minds of its individuals! Have you ever stopped to think that in your mind resides the most potent force in the Universe? It's true! There is practically nothing you can't accomplish if you turn the power of your mind on it. Why so many people fail to utilize even a fraction of what their minds are capable of is the biggest puzzle in the world today. My observation is that it represents nothing short of pure laziness — we tend to drift along in our ruts of complacency, our own little circles of life without bothering to think. And all too soon we reach middle years, our minds completely fallow and withered from disuse just as certainly as our muscles get soft and flabby if not conditioned.

But it's not too late! You can restart that well-oiled dynamo which is your mind even if the rust of time has gathered thick on it.

MIND POWER RESTORES YOUTH

Ralph was a thirty year old man who looked well past his mid-forties. He was overweight but undernourished, completely flab from his double chins down to his tree-trunk legs, malcontent with his job and well into the throes of alcoholism. He couldn't seem to come to grips with physical conditioning or weight control. Diets didn't work and he was convinced they were useless. When I saw him sometime later, it was in the emergency room of a hospital where he'd been brought by his wife. Ralph was in acute alcoholic stupor and extremely ill.

In a couple of days, when the "hairy phase" had passed and he was able to eat and drink without vomiting blood again and his pickled brain had cleared so he could track reasonably well, he asked me a question not uncommon to cases like his: "Doc, what am I going to do? I'm close to losing my job, my wife and family and I'm sick. Can't you do something? Anything?"

"There's not a thing to do for you," I replied, rather sarcastically as I sat down on the edge of his bed. "When you've hit the bottom of the barrel — no, when you've sunk beyond the bottom, you'll be ready to help yourself!" He just looked at me as the words began to sink in. He flew into a rage for a moment, then cooled down a bit.

"You're some doctor!" he growled.

"You're a miserable patient and you're going to die before you're fifty if you keep up this joke you call a life," I replied calmly. "It's *you* that has to decide when you're ready for *me* to help you. When that time comes, let me know."

A few weeks later, Ralph came to see me. He looked better than he had for some time. He asked for the diet, the conditioning routine and wanted to hear again what I'd told him before about his mind. I told him that he had it in *him* to make himself keep up his physical conditioning routines. That he had it in *him* to condition his mind to stay on a diet. And that he had the power in *his* mind to quit the bottle and go on the wagon for good — *if he really wanted to.* At long last, Ralph accepted the power of his mind. Today, Ralph looks younger than his thirty-five years because he mastered his mind's vast resources. You can also master it for a youth transfusion.

STEP THREE: MASTERING YOUR YOUTH CYCLES

The world we live in, the solar system of which we are a part, the galaxy in which our solar system is but a tiny speck and the Universe itself in which our galaxy is almost nothing — all these systems are governed by cycles. So is your body and your mind. You can master them to stay younger.

There are mind cycles, body cycles and mind-body cycles. And hundreds of cycles going on at all times within your organism that you're totally unaware of. There are times when mind will simply not work in accord with body and vice versa. There are times when certain of your cycles need close attention and when their patterns need changing.

YOUTH CYCLES PAY DIVIDENDS FOR THIS MAN

I know a man named Hal who comes as close to anyone in having absolute control over his cycles. He is a successful business man in his early sixties. He could, and often has been taken for about forty-five. How did he do it — just a quirk of Nature? A lucky coincidence? Not at all. He *worked* at it.

Hal never arises in the morning or goes to bed at night without a brief work-out. Sometimes it's only five to ten minutes, sometimes longer, but always as much a part of his day as eating or sleeping. He's been doing this for twenty years! He hasn't tried to make himself look like some muscle-bound ape, he merely keeps his muscles toned as they were when he was younger — no more, no less. If he's unusually tired at the end of a day, he skips the conditioning. He's learned that his body cycles sometimes aren't up to physical exertion at the times usually set aside for it. At other times, Hal tells me he's mentally exhausted — not often, but sometimes. His mind cycles are out of phase. He then gets two to three extra hours of sleep to let his body-mind cycles phase in with the rest of his cycles.

Hal eats an extra snack at mid-morning and mid-afternoon. The snacks consist of carbohydrate (not candy or black coffee) in the form of skim milk, a sweet roll, crackers or yogurt. With this, Hal takes advantage of his blood sugar cycle and keeps a constant supply of vital sugar readily available for his cells to burn as energy. He never suffers from low blood sugar jitters.

Hal never plans important business decisions or meetings during low pressure dips in the weather. He's found that to do so is to invite mistakes. He takes time off from his work and family to do some things *he likes to do.* He's learned how to relax.

Hal enjoys life right along with the things family, business and other duties call for. At sixty, Hal looks, feels and *is* forty-five years young. He will continue to enjoy this state of mind and body as long as he continues to master his youth-building cycles. Plan today to start copying Hal's successful formula!

STEP FOUR: A CLEAN BILL
OF HEALTH FOR VIGOROUS YOUTH

The last of the four cornerstones of youth is your continued good health. Each one of the preceding three keystones for youth will point you in the direction of sparkling robust health. Some final touches are necessary.

A DOUBLE INDEMNITY IN HEALTH

Once in a while, it's my good fortune to accomplish double benefits when it comes to renewing youth in patients. Such was the case of Louise and her husband Richard. Louise first came to my attention with an acute attack of gall bladder disease at the tender age of thirty-eight. It started just like most such trouble does with bloating and pain about an hour after a meal, increasing in intensity and radiating around to the back and the right shoulder blade. This was soon followed by a two or three degree rise in temperature and nausea with vomiting of bile. Louise had had these attacks before and had been warned of her classical "fair, fat and forty" appearance generally associated with gall bladder trouble. She failed to heed the warning. This time, she ended up in the hospital with intravenous feeding, continuous stomach suction through a tube for two days and a very miserable illness.

I visited her one evening as the acute phase was leveling off and found her husband in the room visiting her. I'd never seen him before, but Richard was a man of forty-one, with sparse, balding gray hair, dark circles beneath his eyes and about sixty-five pounds too much weight. A pair of prematurely aged young people, each contributing in his way to the "downfall" of the other!

Both these people had enough of ill-health and feeling like they were eighty. Both started on muscle conditioning, dieting controls and cycle controls. Louise came down from 180 to 120 pounds in about nine months. She became a new, younger woman full of pep and able to keep up physically with any man. She found out what things in her diet were most apt to upset her gall bladder. She regarded such foods taboo from that time forward. Since X-rays revealed no gall stones, surgery was prevented and Louise will probably never need it if she continues to practice her "youthifying." Having regained her youthful outlook on life in general, Louise has become a model mother to her youngsters who were rather on their own before Louise's change.

Ralph, spurred and encouraged by his wife's progress, trimmed off his flab as well and now has 168 pounds of well-toned muscle on his five foot eleven frame. He learned how to stop removing the natural oils from his skin and hair and how to condition it. His hair is thick and vigorous now and though the gray is still there, the thick healthy hair covering the bald spots has taken ten years off Richard's appearance. His facial toning-up exercises have successfully unpacked the bags around his eyes and the dark sickly appearing circles have virtually disappeared with facial isometrics.

Both these very happy youthful people have added twenty useful, healthful and invigorating years to what would have been misery, sickness and an early demise had they continued to let their health run down the drain. You can learn from Richard and Louise. Your health is precious — take care of it for life's sake!

YOUNG NERVES AND ORGANS NEED ENERGY

It's disheartening to see youth just drifting away. Fading without a fight. And it's so needless because the spark that ignites the fires of youth is so easily struck. Rick, a young man of twenty-two, illustrates what I mean.

Rick was a hippie, a member of the acid and beads crowd. A drop-out. And a dismal sight for all his talk of love and peace When I first caught sight of him, I estimated he was at least forty years old. How right I was in some respects!

I first came in contact with this bearded wreck of a man in the medical unit of a mental hospital. He'd come into the hospital with an acute schizophrenic break. He was psychotic — quite mad, in other words, thanks to drugs, loss of identity and strange people around him who couldn't have cared less.

When he first came to the medical unit, having at least been withdrawn from several drugs including LSD, "speed" (the hippie lingo for amphetamines) and marijuana, he was only a shell of a man — thin, so nervous he couldn't sit still or hold his hands steady enough to light a cigarette, and so fatigued he couldn't walk a hundred feet without running out of breath. He'd given up. Thrown in the towel. The final drop-out — from life.

And what had brought him to the medical unit? Someone noticed the whites of his eyes were yellow, and he was beginning to complain of a severe belly ache. Rick was coming down with infectious hepatitis, probably from a dirty needle he'd used to "shoot a little speed." This might be just enough to do him in. Permanently!

But Rick had a little something going for him. He'd gotten off the drugs and in doing so, was beginning to give just a little attention to what was going on around him for a change. He was at least able to complain about his belly ache — something he wouldn't have done a month before.

I watched Rick improve. Slowly at first, because he had to be talked into every bite of food, every glass of nourishment. At first, of course, there were the days of intravenous feeding to deliver pure energy in the form of sugar to his vital structures. Without it, he would certainly succumb. As his liver inflammation subsided over a time, his appetite returned, but not before he'd lost another thirty pounds. At the height of his illness, Rick got down to eighty-nine pounds though he was six feet tall!

When his jaundice began to clear, Rick was put on some muscle toning exercises. He couldn't stand much at first, but for a couple of minutes every day, twice a day, he was literally forced to strain a few muscles. After three weeks, he settled down to the fact that we weren't going to let up so he took off with the conditioning on his own. Soon, he built up his toning time to five minutes three times a day. His body then began to cry out for protein and carbohydrates — to rebuild his wasted muscles and restore his damaged liver cells. Rick got lean meat twice a day and protein supplements between meals and at bedtime. In addition, he poured down at least three rich egg nogs a day and ate four regular meals.

Rick learned about cycles — how to control natural rhythms between body and mind, how to see to it that his mineral cycles, his sugar cycles and his organ cycles were kept in harmony through regular toning, proper diet and mind control. For the first time in some years, Rick began to show an interest in learning. His days in the college he'd attended were sadly wasted, but he picked up where he quit and churned along at a rapid clip. Within another six weeks, he'd thrown off any desire for drugs and was eager to get back to school.

As he put it to me, "You know, things really seem different now. Life's become a challenge. I don't feel the need to be a drag — I want to do something about what the others are saying is wrong with our society."

I think this last statement is noteworthy — wanting to do something — how tough it is to get to this state! How difficult and impossible it seems. Yet, there is a way to ignite the spark.

Rick did it and finally recovered those lost years from neglect of his organism. His liver returned to normal size and will remain there if he stays away from alcohol and drugs. His mind is now working for him rather than against him — he learned to control it while in the hospital. And his nerves and organs are functioning at top efficiency again. His weight was back up to 155 when he left the hospital and his muscles were trim and solid. The last word I had was that he will graduate from college this summer and plans to do graduate work.

INVOLUTIONAL MELANCHOLIA REVERSED

Isn't it strange that some lives must be suddenly thrown into limbo just because the halfway point is at hand? And the odd part of it is that most of the trouble that begins at or near menopause in women is largely conditioned, largely brought about by the expectation of doom at mid-life!

Eva was such a woman. Her menstrual periods began to taper off about the age of forty-one. They hadn't stopped, just began to taper. And to Eva, this spelled the end of everything. She began to mope around. Began to become suspicious of people — to question the motives of those around her, even her family. Soon she had them all working "against her" and "not caring." Eva's reaction to all this fancied conspiracy was to withdraw gradually from life. She refused to go out of her house. Refused to have people in. Became angry when she saw her family having fun or enjoying themselves — behaved like a child to insure their fun was short-lived.

Over the following three years, Eva began to eat as a defense against the gnawing trouble inside her mind — when she got upset or nervous, she ate. The more she ate, the flabbier she got. She also developed dry, scaly skin, thin frayed hair and lost her sexual drive completely. It was at this station that her family appealed to a mental health center for help.

Fortunately, Eva's "involutional melancholia," another way of saying reaction to the menopause, hadn't progressed to the point of no return. Through the newer group therapy contacts at the center, Eva began to take an interest in her surroundings and in the people around her as humans trying to help rather than plotting against her. Short term antidepressant therapy using drugs helped raise her from the sea of despair and help-lessness.

At this point, she began her "youthifying" trip — she began to unload those years from her badly treated organism.

The first step was to lose fifty-three extra pounds she had added to an already stretched frame. This she did by limiting her diet to less calories than she actually needed every day to get through her various activities. Eva lost ten pounds the first month. Next she started her physical conditioning routines. She started with ten minutes twice a day. A few isometrics at first, then one calisthenic sit-up for her abdomen which had turned into a mass of flab — then another added to this in about two weeks. Within a month, Eva was doing twenty-five minutes of exercises twice a day. Another ten pounds went off and finely toned, lithe muscles replaced those she'd allowed to waste away.

And Eva learned mind-body cycle control as well as anyone I've seen. She learned that she could control her mood through auto-suggestion. She began to understand what the things were that depressed her. She learned to react to these attitudes differently by concentrating at intervals during the day and at bedtime — she cycled her mind to think of other things — creative work, physical exertion, concern about her family and friends — all these and more replaced the "sorry for me" thoughts that formerly made her renounce life. In two more months, she was off drugs.

Within six months, Eva transformed herself into a living example of what can be done given a little help, a little insight and a lot of stimulus to help oneself. She peeled off about twenty years from her frame. She not only looked but *was* younger for the effort. At present, Eva is at work helping others come along the road she herself traveled. And she's doing a whale of a job at it!

THE ROAD BACK

Is it a foregone conclusion that natural aging must preclude youth? That senility sets in at sixty and progresses from that point on! It is, IF it's allowed to do so! That it isn't necessarily something that one must simply endure is demonstrated day in and day out in the geriatrics units of mental health centers around the country.

I'm thinking about a lady named Nell, age seventy. Nell, it seems, began her trouble while staying with one of her married sons. No one could remember just when it started. Maybe with a sharp word of criticism here, a crying spell there. Anyway, it had happened. Things got so bad at the home that it was decided that the best thing for Nell was a nursing home. So, off to the nursing home went Nell. Much, I might add, against her wishes, though something, it was obvious, had to be done.

From here, things got worse, indeed. She was mad at everybody and everything. She flew into a rage at the slightest provocation, and often with no provocation at all. She quarrelled with her roommates (she went through several), she quarrelled with the staff. Even with herself alone in her room. The staff, harried and overworked, and without time, really, to try and understand what was making Nell act up, reacted as best they could. Soon, they "just couldn't handle her" any longer. She was transferred to a mental hospital.

When Nell arrived at the hospital she was a living example of "a woman scorned." Her wrath had no limits. She threatened mayhem to the first to touch her. She was dirty and unkempt. She sat alone and wouldn't eat.

By gently persuading Nell that she was, indeed, going to behave herself, by getting her off her chair and out of her room, making her move again, things began to look up. Her appetite returned and she found herself being friendly to others again. Gradually, she was worked into a more vigorous routine of activity — long walks on and off the grounds, trips to the occupational therapy department for activities such as weaving, clay modeling and the like, parties given by and attended by her ward mates and so on. Very soon, Nell was a changed person. She became pleasant. She had no more rages or tirades. She became the epitome of cleanliness and practiced excellent personal hygiene without prompting.

In a short time, she was ready to leave the hospital. Her son and daughter-in-law, amazed by her change, wanted, even begged her to come back to their home. It was at this point that Nell made what I consider a masterful decision. She said, "No, I don't think that would be the best idea. You know, us older folks have a little different way of thinking than you younger ones. Oh, I'm not saying it's bad, but that's the way it is. I think I'll go to a nursing home again. Maybe not the same one as before, but one where I can help some of the others adjust." What insight! What remarkable good sense!

Senility? Certainly not. Wisdom! And a good deal more than most of her juniors!

YOUTH HIGHWAY OR RUT OF FEAR?

Often, I think of a man I knew named Mike. Mike was fifty years old, looked sixty and acted seventy. Why? Mike had become a "cardiac cripple." He'd suffered his heart attack at the age of forty-nine, and was literally spending most of his waking hours in dread of the second.

Mike was in self-exile at home. Before his coronary, he'd been a highly successful insurance salesman. Had a good outlook on life, a good physique, was a vital, robust person with plenty on the ball. But not anymore. He felt that if he weren't an invalid, he'd die any moment from another coronary. Actually, he was setting the stage for death from yet another cause entirely. Namely, deterioration by fear.

When he'd spent his customary three weeks in the hospital, Mike was advised to take it easy at first — no more exercise than was necessary to get around the house, strict cholesterol-free diet, take his medicines regularly and appear at the hospital every week or two for blood checks to see if his medicines were doing their jobs properly.

Mike followed his instructions to the limit. The only thing was that Mike developed a morbid fear of having to go through it all over again — perhaps with fatal results. He must prevent this at any cost, he thought. And the only way to do it was to keep absolutely quiet. No unnecessary movement, no straining, no stress.

All of which was good for a time. But Mike wouldn't give it up. Efforts to get him off his front porch were futile. He insisted on stark quiet — had the telephone removed. Had the television taken to the basement. Took a nap every two or three hours. Deterioration!

When I first saw Mike, he was beginning to have pains in both his legs. As the story came out, I realized why. He was developing phlebitis in the veins of his legs because he never used them for anything but to sit or to go to the bathroom or kitchen for more sitting. His elimination system had gone to pot as well and he found it necessary to use laxatives constantly to keep his bowels moving. And his thinking had been affected. The old Mike — the outward-going guy thinking of others more than himself — was submerged in self-pity and fear. This was going to be tough.

Since Mike's physician had become ill and was hospitalized himself, I took the bull by the horns. I went to Mike's house one evening to check on his phlebitis. Instead of the usual greetings and conversation, I said, "Well, Mike, how long are you going to let Rita do your dirty work for you?"

There followed a surprised look, followed by a scowl, followed by the explanation, "What are you talking about? Why, I'm . . . a sick man. What do you mean?"

"I mean exactly what I said. When are you going to start getting the lead out?" An open mouth and scowl again.

"Are you crazy? Why, Doctor Manfreed said . . ."

"I know what he said. But he said it eight months ago. What about now, Mike?"

When Mike got over the shock, I managed to convince him of one thing. He had to get off his duff and get moving. Get back into the stream. I was able to convince him he could look and feel closer to forty than his present sixtyish and that his heart would tell him in plenty of time to slow down if he overdid it.

I showed him how to use his mind to condition himself for the next step. Just before dozing off to sleep, he was to concentrate on being active. Put everything else out of his mind and repeat over and over, "I will be active tomorrow." Soon Mike was walking around the block. He was doing three, then six blocks. Next Mike started a few simple isometrics — the soft exercises. He was surprised. He could actually exercise without dire consequences! He peeled off eighteen pounds over the next two months and began to show a glimmer of that old Mike again. He contacted his company, and was again pleasantly surprised to find his old job open — with help enough to take some of the old pressure off his daily chores.

Mike lost his anxiety about his heart. He lost his phlebitis. He has gained an entirely new outlook on life that has made him younger. Today, Mike can do anything he wants physically without angina — heart pain that signals too much exertion. He hasn't climbed any mountains or taken up skiing yet, but he doesn't really need to tempt fate that much now. He *knows* he can lead a normal, youthful, healthy life again.

CHAPTER SUMMARY

1. There are four main steps to take today for restoring your youth. Practice them conscientiously, faithfully, religiously for the continuing restoration of youth.
    A. A vigorous body with youth hide, a resilient frame and smoothly working innards is achieved through conditioning and weight control.
    B. A dynamic, youthful mind is achieved by tapping the reservoirs of power lying dormant in your brain.
    C. The control of body, mind, chemical, physical and weather cycles will help you establish permanent youth.
    D. Total health means total youth. You can help recapture youth by regaining your health.

2

How You Can Regain a Glowing Youthful Figure Through Simple Weight Control

It used to be thought that fat people were happy people. Would that it were so, but nothing could be further from the truth. Fat people are unhappy. The reason is that they are subject to so many ills, aches and pains that they age two to three times faster than normal. I'd like to show you how easy it is to avoid this unnecessary aging through control of your weight.

You need to know how to peel off useless flab and how to keep it peeled off for a permanently youthful figure. It really isn't as difficult as you may have been led to believe, or as you, yourself, may have made the task in the past only to give it up as a hopeless cause.

There are a few pearls that will help you lose weight and keep it lost once you've come down. I'll talk about these in this section. Many people tend to blame outside influences of absolutely no consequence on their weight problems. I want to point these out and show them up for what they are: — self deluding imagination. Still other people feel that to lose weight means to take potent and dangerous drugs. This idea needs to be laid to rest immediately and permanently, and I'll show you how to do it.

Finally, a good many of you will have a rather hopeless attitude toward your weight problem because you're going through or have already gone through menopause, and you have the idea that weight gain is a necessary evil that goes along with the "change of life." I want to show you why this isn't true and how you can restore youth at or beyond menopause with weight control.

EXCESS WEIGHT IS DANGEROUS TO YOUTH!

The following is a partial list of serious diseases brought on or materially worsened by excess weight:

Coronary heart disease	Stroke	Gall Stones
Hyptertension (high blood pressure)	Blood vessel degeneration	Varicose veins
Liver Disease	Diabetes	Arthritis

Among these disease states are the top killers and cripplers of Americans today. Doesn't it make good sense that avoiding them means not only better health but more youthful living for you as well? Certainly it does. You can literally add years to your body by getting rid of the common denominator in all the above diseases: *by getting that weight down to reasonable levels and keeping it there!*

And what is reasonable? Use the following rule of thumb to see whether your weight is reasonable:

MEN: Between five and six feet tall (without shoes) = 100 pounds plus six pounds for each inch over five feet.
Between six and seven feet tall (without shoes) = 173 pounds plus seven pounds for each inch beyond six feet.

WOMEN: Same as men except add four pounds for each inch beyond five feet.

This rule assumes that your frame — your bones and muscles — are of medium size. For light frames, ten to fifteen pounds must be subtracted from this ideal weight; for heavy frames, the same may be added to this ideal weight. A good way to tell about your frame is by your shirt or blouse size. It's well to remember that you will live longer and stay younger if you carry about 10 percent less than your ideal weight after age forty years.

STARTING YOUR YOUTH DIET TODAY

Of all the fads and fancy frills on our American scene, those concerned with dieting are the most numerous and most complicated and seem to me the most useless of all. It's really simple to lose weight. All you need to do is to burn up more calories than you take in each day until your body burns up the excess fat stored in your body. From then on, you need only take in roughly the amount of energy you burn up, and your weight will remain steady. And you will remain younger!

THE SIX POINT DIET

The following is all you need to know to lose weight safely:

1. Tonight, when you sit down to supper, stop all activity after you've filled your plate with its usual portions of whatever you are eating. Now do the "calorie slicing maneuver": divide all the carbohydrate foods into four sections and put back in the serving dish three of these sections. Do the same with fat foods and return half to the serving dish. If you're still hungry, make up the difference by eating protein food.

   The same should be done at every meal. A table at the end of this book gives a list of which foods are carbohydrate, which are protein and which are fats. If you do this simple procedure at each meal, *you cannot help but lose weight!* No fads. No fancy jimcracks. No tricks to play on yourself!

2. *Eat smaller meals* and have a snack between meals at mid-morning, mid-afternoon and bedtime. Use rule 1 with snacks, too. You're trying to shrink your stomach so that it doesn't hit you with an appetite "like a horse" all throughout the day. The way to shrink it is to put less inside it and to stem the appetite pangs that plague you.

3. *Eliminate entirely* the following foods from your diet until your weight is where you want it:

Butter	Egg yolk (white O.K.)	Candy	*All* baked goods
Cream	Sugar (sub-stitutes O.K.)	Pop	Cooking oils
Salad dressings	Syrup from canned fruit		75 percent of your booze
Gravy	All desserts		

Years of trial and error have proven beyond all reasonable doubt that *none* of the above foods are compatible with losing weight. Actually, if you never again had a bite or a drop of any of the items from the above list, you'd never miss them! For butter, substitute *margarine*. For cream and whole milk, substitute *skim milk*. For salad dressings, substitute vinegar and herbs. For eggs, substitute meat, cheese, leguminous vegetables (any that grow in a pod like peas and beans). For gravy, substitute the *juices from cooked vegetables.*

4. *Do not eat when you're nervous, upset or moody!* Overeating is natural when you're emotionally involved. Eat with peace and quiet prevailing and after you've cooled down and relaxed. Two or three ounces of Sherry before mealtime is an excellent "tranquillizer."

5. *Do not skip meals* and don't drink black coffee on an empty stomach. Skipping meals invites your stomach to call for three times the usual quantity of food the next meal. Black coffee taken by itself causes low blood sugar with an enormous uncontrollable appetite to follow! Have coffee *with meals*. Use something other than coffee at breaks, or take in some carbohydrate with your coffee (crackers, cookies, toast for example).

6. *Always do physical conditioning when losing weight.* These six steps are all you need to know to diet. You don't even have to know what a calorie is to avoid them. Don't settle for less than fifteen to twenty pounds of weight loss at the end of six weeks on your diet routine. From then on, five to ten pounds a month is fast enough. If you aren't losing at this rate, you've let one or more of the six steps slip — review them again and really tighten down! It will work! Start today to recapture your youthful figure the easy way!

FOUR SECRETS OF WEIGHT STABILIZATION

When you have your weight where you want it, what then? "I'll just gain it all back again" is the lament I hear every day. No you won't! Not if you follow these four guidelines to keep your weight down once you get it under control.

A. Your Nerves and Your Weight

If you haven't already discovered it, you will be like a patient I know named Bill who had the difficult problem of nervous eating. Bill was about sixty-five pounds overweight when I first met him. It was getting to a point where Bill's health demanded weight reduction. He was in the midst of ulcer trouble, had a liver ailment and couldn't walk a hundred feet before being completely winded. He was thirty-two years old and he looked and felt closer to fifty.

Bill swore to me that he didn't overeat. "Why," he said, "I eat like a bird!" I refrained from calling him a liar, but that's just what I thought. Where did all his heft come from? Heaven? Providence? Gland trouble? Even with glandular disturbances, and they're extremely rare, the disturbed glands have to have something to make fat out of — they can't do it from thin air!

It wasn't until later when I talked with Bill's wife that I found out part of Bill's difficulty: it seems he went to the refrigerator three or four times during the course of an evening for "snacks." His "snacks" regularly consisted of helpings of meat with the fat left on, potato chips, bread with butter and jam, and a large portion of whatever there had been for dessert at supper time! An entire meal at every "snack"!

In addition, I found out that what in Bill's eyes was "just a little bit" of food, to most would seem enough for three people. Bill had been fooling himself to the point that *he actually believed he didn't eat very much!*

There were times Bill didn't even know when he wolfed down all this food — he was a nervous wreck and whenever the pressure was on, and this was just about all the time, he would unconsciously go to the larder for something to poke into his stomach. And he could never stop with just a piece of a candy bar. Without realizing it, after the first piece would automatically follow eight or ten more! This was the way Bill lived — a compulsive eater — a "foodoholic," so the speak.

At first, Bill denied all this when I threw it up to him. Instead of fighting him on the issue, I asked him to tell me frankly what it really was that "got to him" so much — what it was that "bugged" him. Then followed the source of Bill's uncontrollable eating habits: he had trouble at his work, was often passed over for promotion and felt inferior and guilty. This problem didn't just start recently. Bill had *always* felt inferior. The method Bill used to offset this very uncomfortable feeling of self-pity and inferiority? He ate — and ate — and ate.

When Bill learned a new method of handling his feelings, for instance that of substituting physical exertion for feelings of hunger, the battle of the bulge was won. Just by substituting another habit — one that was part of a good reducing regime anyway — Bill overcame his inability to hold weight loss. He is slim and trim today, and he has a better understanding of himself for the slight inconvenience he went to in working over his eating habits.

B. Exercise and Holding Your Weight

A while ago in the six point diet program, I left point six unexplained. It's so important that I'm devoting an entire section to it. The neglect of this point is the reason so many people not only have trouble losing weight but keeping their weight down once they manage to reduce.

In talking some time ago with a lady named Irma, neglect of conditioning was brought out quite well. I'd seen her several times before and had started her on a typical weight reduction routine. This was back in the days when even I wasn't convinced (or enlightened) concerning the wisdom of proper physical conditioning and dieting.

"I just can't understand it, doctor. I've done everything you told me, I'm starving myself to death, but I don't get anywhere!" Irma complained. I reviewed my records. Irma hadn't lost more than four pounds in the last ten weeks in spite of her rigid diet. I immediately suspected Irma was another Bill in the case just described. But I knew Irma was a strong-willed person not given much to nervousness. Neither did she prove to be an ice-box raider, nor a "snacker," according to her husband.

Then I began to wonder about her glandular system and whether I'd missed something in the way of disease or slow down in one of her endocrine glands. To verify the question, I checked on her thyroid, adrenal and ovarian glands. They were all working perfectly normally. As we talked further about her everyday life, I discovered an interesting point: Irma began to have weight problems at exactly the same time she was married. And her husband once remarked that Irma would never suffer what his mother had, namely, to slave around the house and work her "fingers to the bone." This was the clue! Irma was literally gathering flab and useless fat and aging in the process, because she never did anything that even resembled physical activity.

The next thing I did was put Irma on three physical work-out sessions every day. Slow and easy at first — five to six minutes until she got used to using her soft flabby muscles again. When she became accustomed to it, I increased the time until she was spending fifteen to twenty minutes three times a day. She joined a health club in addition to her home sessions.

This routine plus her dieting started the pounds shedding like water off a duck's back. The first week, Irma lost seven pounds; the second week, six more; the third week, nine more. In the span of six months, Irma lost seventy pounds while during the previous six months she'd managed to lose only about eight pounds!

C. Alcohol and Your Weight

Your alcohol intake may be slight, great, or none at all. If you're like millions of Americans, it is "moderate." At any rate, alcohol does pile up the calories and may cause what might be an easy weight shedding process to become a nightmare. And it may be a reason that you always gain back what weight your good efforts lose for you!

A most remarkable example of this point comes to mind. A man named Rod, whom I'd known for years, responded to weight control programs almost overnight — he could lose ten, twenty, even thirty pounds in about six weeks whenever he wanted. When he'd gone through about six such episodes, each time coming back to me for diet instructions, etc., I began to wonder about this "shrinking-expanding" man. What in the world was going on, I wondered, to cause Rod's weight to come and go like the tides?

When he came to me the last time for advice on his weight problem, I noticed his very red (plethoric) face, the prominent tiny skin veins and an enlarged liver. Rod was an alcoholic! Oh, Rod didn't admit it. In fact, he vehemently denied it when I suggested it to him. "Aw, Doc," he said, "I never drink more than a couple in the evening." Rod's "couple" consisted, I found out later, of two large tumblers with the equivalent of four shots of whiskey in each one! He also neglected to mention that on week-ends and at parties (he and his wife entertained a lot in the course of Rod's sales position) going home completely polluted was rather commonplace.

Of course, Rod was headed for an early grave and he was digging it himself. Everytime Rod put down a "couple" in the evening, he was adding about 2000 calories to his system — when you are trying to lose weight, about half this amount is as much as you need during the entire day!

Rod needed his alcohol. Without going into the psychoanalysis necessary to find out why, I managed to steer him away from excess booze by getting him to *admit* he had a problem. Without this, any therapy where booze is concerned is futile. When he was able to face this fact, Rod was eventually able to substitute physical conditioning and a hobby for his alcohol. When this was accomplished, Rod had no more weight problems.

D. Controlling Weight Cycles

Your body cycles and how to control them will be the subject of section five. At this point, you need to know that they do, indeed, affect your success with weight control.

Jane had such a problem with cycles. In this case, her menstrual cycle was the culprit. Jane had gained weight steadily since age 13 years, the age at which her monthly periods started. She'd never been able to effectively control her weight gain, and she was convinced her "glands were haywire." She'd been on thyroid extract, taken just "in case my thyroid was slow," but it hadn't done a thing except to make her jumpy and jittery and actually added to her weight gain problem. She'd also been placed on estrogen hormone therapy. At the tender age of twenty-eight, Jane needed estrogen hormones about as much as she needed another head.

In talking with Jane, she told me that every month, about a week before her period started, she got nervous, easily upset and developed an enormous appetite. This went on until her flow started, then the urge for food stopped. But it happened every month, month in and month out. Any gains she made in dieting for three weeks of the month was offset by the losses during this frustrating fourth week. The consequence was that Jane was now about eighty-five pounds overweight!

The answer to Jane's problem was fairly easy after it became clear that what she needed was cycle control. First, Jane was given physical conditioning along with dieting *to be intensified at double the rate during the week before her period was to start.* All drugs she'd been on were stopped, and a mild sedative prescribed *to be used only during the week before her periods.* It took Jane about twenty-eight months to come down to normal, but she made it. She looks ten years younger and has never felt better in her life. Incidentally, I took her off the mild sedative after only ten weeks. She didn't need it any longer once she mastered control of her nerves and she could see the results of concentrated effort directed at cycle control.

THROW WEIGHT CONTROL
DRUGS IN THE TRASH CAN

I've raised the question of drugs in relation to weight control. Appetite control drugs generally are *the most useless group of drugs on the market today!* Their side-effects are so numerous and detract so much from the problems at hand that I never use them, and neither should you. All such drugs are stimulants, they make nervous wrecks of you and they keep you awake nights. As if this weren't enough, most of these drugs are *habit-forming.* They are psychologically as well as physiologically addicting in some cases. They are the same group of drugs that many youngsters today are "shooting" into their bloodstreams in the form of "speed" and "crystal."

I examined a patient named Phyllis recently who landed in a mental hospital having taken such drugs too much and too long. She had an acute psychotic break and isn't over it yet!

If you need drugs to reduce, you aren't ready. You can get ready by mastering the next two sections.

SO YOU THINK YOUR GLANDS ARE AT FAULT?

Since endocrine glands, about which we'll talk more later, are blamed more for people being overweight than any other one thing, I present the following table for you to check out. If you do not have all the symptoms and signs, then your glands are *not at fault*. If you do have them, you should check with your doctor.

GLAND	SIGNS OF UNDERACTIVITY	SYMPTOMS
Thyroid	Dry skin, dry and brittle frayed hair.	Lassitude, hair falling out.
	Mental disorders.	Inability to think properly.
	Menstrual overactivity.	Mania and/or with-drawal into a shell. Excessive menstrual bleeding.
	Constipation, chronic stomach and bowel trouble and anemia.	Fatigue, short-windedness.
	Fluid retention.	"Stove-pipe" legs and arms.
Adrenals	Fat pads back of neck. "Moon" face and plethora.	"Buffalo hump" and round shiny face.
	Pounding headaches and chest pains.	High blood pressure.
	Menstrual cessation.	Rapid heart beat.
	Fluid retention.	Sexual decline.
	Weight gain on chest and abdomen: none on extremities.	Edema (fluid in tissues).

MENOPAUSE MYTH SLAIN

A lady I call "Catherine the Great" illustrates well the myth of so-called Menopause Obesity. It has become a watchword among far too many women that the onset of menopause automatically brings on fat and the decline of life in general. Actually nothing could be further from the truth as Catherine's case will show.

Catherine was forty-nine years old, had always enjoyed good health and was about a year past menopause. This is to say, her menstrual periods stopped when she was forty-eight years old. She was five feet six inches tall and weighed 231 pounds! A walking blimp. When I saw her for the first time, she complained of shortness of breath on the slightest physical exertion, palpitations of her heart, headaches, bowel trouble, unusually severe constipation, dropsy (collection of fluid in the lower legs and ankles) and she said she was depressed most of the time. On further talking, Catherine told me she couldn't seem to get along with her kids and her husband had threatened to walk out on her. She was a very miserable woman.

I asked Catherine if she ever considered her tremendous obesity as a reason for all her familial discord — as a reason, and a good one, that her husband might want to "walk out" on her. "But doctor," she exclaimed, "I've just entered menopause! There's nothing I can do about the way I look." I just stared at her for a few minutes and finally replied, "If you can't, then I'm afraid there's nothing anybody else can do for you either."

The chief reason for Catherine's "greatness" of weight was that she had been so thoroughly convinced that she was finished as a woman that she let herself develop into a walking Sherman tank!

When Catherine began to realize that it was *she* who was responsible for any failure she might have been as wife and mother and that she had it in her to come out of her shell, she recovered.

Under diet restriction, she began trimming pounds. This was helped and spurred along by physical conditioning. In two years, Catherine The Great changed into something vastly different. Her weight dropped to 135, a loss of ninety-six pounds! She was totally unrecognizable as the same blimp who walked into my office two years before. Catherine is living proof of the myth of "menopause fat" being a necessary evil in women past forty-five!

CHAPTER SUMMARY

1. The most vicious cripplers and killers of Americans today are caused and attended by excess weight. You can regain youth and robust health by heading these conditions off with weight reduction starting today.

2. Dieting is usually made overly complicated and weird diet fads have their day from time to time, but there are six rules of thumb for effective dieting for weight control. Once your weight is controlled, the four steps to keeping it that way are easily made a part of your youth-building.

3. Weight control is 99.99 percent accomplished without drugs of any kind. Your glands aren't at fault with your weight problem. Discover youth today by forgetting glands and drugs and remembering simple principles of nutrition.

4. Menopause does not mean the end of your life. Youth begins at forty-five. Don't let yourself believe the myths surrounding menopause.

3

How to Condition Your Body for Youthful Strength and Vigor

You're now ready to start restoring youth to your body's frame. This frame consists of bony skeleton, muscles and connective tissues. In building a youthful body, your frame may be compared to the foundation, joints and roof of a house. If any one of these essential items is defective in a building, it collapses. You don't want this to happen to you because if it does, youth flies out the window. I want to show you how you can restore youthful litheness to your bones and muscles.

Not only can you invigorate your frame and keep it young, but you can take advantage of the "built-in" bonus that goes along with conditioning. Not only do your blood vessels, glands and organs derive renewed youthful potency from conditioning, your mind is likewise stimulated to vigorous creative activity through proper physical conditioning! I want to explain how to get these premiums from physical conditioning and keep on getting them the rest of your life.

DIET PLUS EXERCISE DOES THE TRICK

You've seen in the previous section how the supposedly difficult job of shedding flab can be made easy. I want you to memorize this point: There is no effective dieting without conditioning and no conditioning without fat-control. The reason is simple. You've seen what happens to muscles and skeleton and connective tissue when useless fat is allowed to collect. Now that you're in the process of taking that fat down, *it's important to restore muscle tone to prevent that sagging, aging "middle-aged" spread!*

MAN LOSES WEIGHT, REMAINS BLOB

Jim, a man of forty-three years, started a weight-losing routine and did a very good job of it. He told me he'd always been a walking pork barrel and was sick and tired of it. He listened intently as I recounted the principles of the previous section to him. He had a determined will and had rather large muscles on his five foot eleven inch frame. His trouble lay in the fact that his weight fluctuated between 220 and 235 pounds.

Jim had been an athlete in high school and college. He lettered in both wrestling and football. Now Jim's frame was of the heavy type — he was wide and large-boned, and his muscles were large. Using the rule of thumb listed in the previous section, Jim's ideal weight should be 100 pounds + sixty-six pounds (6 x 11 inches in height) + twenty pounds (the maximum addition for heavy frame) = 186 pounds. As a matter of fact, he recalled that in his prime in college, his weight never exceeded 190 pounds and was usually 185 pounds when wrestling. It had been some years since Jim weighed in at his ideal level!

I reminded Jim that he wasn't playing football or wrestling anymore. He was no longer keeping in shape by adhering to a tight daily physical conditioning routine. But Jim thought he could regain his youthful drive and figure again simply by shedding the flab, about forty-five to fifty pounds of it, he'd accumulated over the years. This was Jim's first mistake. His second was in believing that he would recover all his lost zip and go-power by reducing.

Jim reduced all right. He lost forty pounds in about six months by sticking with his diet. But as he lost his weight, the sagging, unsightly muscles, heretofore hidden by his excess fat, began to show through. He sagged like an aging weather-beaten tent, and he felt his energy waning with each passing week.

As a result, Jim was a very disappointed man when I saw him later on, forty pounds lighter, but almost completely "do-less."

I had Jim undress when next I saw him in the office. Then I had him stand in front of a full length mirror. "Look at yourself," I said. "Look at that face! How could you ever let those chins below your chin develop? Look at your posture! Slouched and slumped like a man of eighty — where is your pride?" He stood there a minute, gazing at the sorry looking sight the mirror reflected back. "You know, Doc," he finally replied, "You're right! It can't be done. You can't just get rid of fat and turn out anything but a dismal heap of jelly."

Now Jim was getting the picture. Here was a former athlete, and a good one, reduced to a quivering shapeless mass. Why? Because he let himself slip out of condition and hadn't bothered to regain it!

I started Jim on the following routine:

1. First thing in the morning on arising:
   a. Sit-ups. Fifteen at first, increasing one or two each week up to forty or fifty. Lying flat on back on the floor, hands clasped behind neck; legs outstretched and kept straight; and no bending legs when "sitting up"; touching left elbow to right knee then the reverse at next "sit-up." *Stomach muscles to accomplish all "sitting" pull.*
   b. Rocking Horse. Lying on stomach on floor; legs bent at knee and ankles grasped by hands. Rearing motion backward back arched, legs pulling arms and body backward. Then frontward thrust, pulling with arms and body frontward and "rocking" on belly so that chin on floor and legs up in the air. Five at first, increasing one or two a week until fifteen or twenty.
2. Last thing at night before going to bed:
   a. Push-ups. Ten at first, increasing one or two each week up to thirty or forty and done as rapidly as possible. Flat on stomach on floor, legs outstretched and kept straight, palms of hands on floor just beneath shoulders with arms bent at elbows. Arms, chest and shoulders *to do all "pushing up" motion:* feel pull in back of upper arms, front of chest and in shoulders.

I asked Jim to take as much time as he needed at first to get through the sessions — I cautioned him *not* to be in a hurry until he felt his strength and vigor returning after a couple of weeks. Later, I told him to begin to add speed to his conditioning — to see, for instance, how many sit-ups he could do in a minute and a half; then in one minute.

I also instructed him to walk at least a mile and a half every day over the noon hour or at any time during the day he could work it in. It could be in two or three separate "walks" if he found it easier, but to go the distance each day. In about a month, double this distance then triple it later on. This, I added, *in addition* to any walking he might do at work.

In three months, Jim was literally a new man! When he came to the office, I imagined the speciman I saw was very close to the young wrestler and football player of twenty years ago! Jim told me he never felt better, that he was doing even more conditioning than prescribed because it felt so good to be in shape once again and that he felt like he was twenty-five rather than his forty-three years. Jim was alive with youthful zip and verve. He told me he'd been having fresh new ideas his boss liked so well that a promotion was soon to be forthcoming. Jim also eventually lost twenty more pounds and was at ideal weight for the first time in twenty years!

Profit from Jim's case. Start your conditioning routine today and keep it a part of your life from now on!

WOMAN EXERCISES BACK TO
YOUTH AND HEALTH

Another patient I know named Helen had just the opposite problem of Jim's. She thought she could condition herself without having to go to the trouble of dieting away her mountain of flab as well. She lived to regret it!

Helen had already started her conditioning before I ever saw her as a patient. She and some of her friends thought it would be nice to start doing something about their fat problems. Somehow, they got the mistaken idea that conditioning would be the last and complete answer to restoring youth to their aging bodies.

So Helen and friends started jogging and swimming and bicycle riding and a number of other things designed to rejuvenate themselves. And it probably would have worked were it not for the fact that one day, while jogging, Helen overdid. She ran to far, too fast, with too much — 214 pounds on a five foot four frame. She collapsed and was delivered to the emergency room of a local hospital where I happened to be the first to see her.

Helen had gone into acute cardiac decompensation, another way of saying that she demanded more pumping action of her heart than her heart muscle could possibly respond with. The result was that the muscle fibers of her heart would no longer contract to pump the blood to her circulation so her circulation stopped, or at least slowed down to the point that her lungs and tissues became congested with blood. Helen recovered rather uneventfully from this episode and while visiting her in the hospital a few days later, I asked her if she didn't think that reducing her vast weight would have been a more safe thing to start before so much physical conditioning. "Yes," she answered, "it would have. But I've tried all those diets and the pills — none of them work. I get so frustrated and angry with diets that I didn't want to go through another one."

I advised Helen that she was about to become a diabetic along with the rest of her physical shortcomings. I told her she'd arrived at a point where she had no choice. She *must* lose weight or suffer the consequences of serious progressive disease. So Helen did lose weight. The digitalis and other drugs she'd been put on to correct her heart failure were gradually diminished and finally stopped altogether. Helen lost forty-five pounds in the span of about seven months! At this time, I broached the subject of conditioning with Helen. "What?" she exclaimed. "Me exercise again? Are you kidding, doctor?"

"No, I'm not kidding," I replied. "What's more, I want you to start it now and keep it up just as faithfully as you've been keeping up your weight losing."

She looked aghast. The mere thought of going through what her last conditioning effort produced was too much for Helen to swallow. But when she found that her routine didn't include jogging, swimming or bicycle riding, at least at this time, she began to listen to reason. Here is the routine I put Helen on.

1. First thing in the morning on arising:
   a. Stomach isometrics. Standing up straight, sucking in stomach as much as possible, chest thrown out, breath sucked clear in. Holding this "sucked-in" position until quivering of abdominal muscles starts, then letting up "sucked-in" position and pulling downward with

stomach muscles so that they bend you over at waist — tightening them down as hard as possible. Repeat cycle five-ten-twenty times, increasing number with passage of time.

b. Arm and chest isometrics. Standing up straight, grasping hands in front of your abdomen with fingers curled over those of opposite side, pulling in opposite directions with arms, slowly bending elbows toward sides until elbows touch sides, then pushing in with elbows as hard as possible while continuing to grasp hands in manner described. Push against sides until chest muscle felt to contract (pectorals are large main chest muscles behind nipples in both males and females). Repeat cycle as many times as possible.

2. Last thing at night before retiring:

a. Leg isometrics. Leaning against a dresser or other support, grasping left ankle with left hand, bending leg at knee to do so. Bending leg at knee forcibly in opposite direction (as though trying to straighten it out). Make back muscles arch back as well. Do same with opposite leg and hand. Repeat cycle until fatigued.

b. Hip swing. Using similar support as for a., swing right leg backward as far as hip muscle (buttock) will pull it without bending leg at knee. Now swing forward in same fashion, no bending at knee. Later on, tie weight such as ordinary iron or book to lower leg or foot and repeat. Do same with opposite leg. Increase number and distance of swings to tolerance.

In spite of the fact that Helen lost over seventy-five pounds over the next sixteen months she did *not* have breasts sagging down to her navel; she did *not* have loose flabby skin hanging over her pubis like an apron; she did *not* have sagging floppy buttocks that caused her to appear like a waddling duck; and she didn't have any further trouble with her heart. Why? Simple. Her heart did not have to pump blood through miles of blood vessels and pounds of useless flab anymore! And continuing her routines after her weight loss is her insurance *that she will never have to worry about her heart again because she's conditioning it as well as her other muscles!* Of course, now that Helen has come down to within five pounds of her ideal weight, she no longer has any troubles doing jogging, swimming, bicycle riding and a host of other physical activities that she thoroughly enjoys.

PROPER CONDITIONING ADDS
YOUTH TO YOUR FRAME

Conditioning is easy! All you need to do is to try it once — for just three weeks, and you'll feel so much better, feel so much more robust, that you'll feel "naked for the day" if you skip your conditioning!

It's especially interesting if you do "your own thing" with conditioning. Consider the following points.

Isometrics

An isometric exercise is one in which one group of muscles is 'pitted' against the same group on the opposite side of your body. If you grasp your hands with curled fingers, as in Helen's routine given a minute ago, and pull in the opposite direction, you're doing an isometric. If you *push* the palms of your two hands together, your arms elevated in front of your chest, elbows bent at right angles, you're doing an isometric — using just the opposite set of muscles as in *pulling* in the same position. Isometrics condition *stamina* into muscles.

You can do an isometric exercise with virtually any set of muscles you have. All you need to do is "set" the opposing muscles and pull, push, stretch or strain the muscle you want to condition. A rule of thumb is: When doing isometrics, always give as much attention to the opposing muscles as you do with the others. For instance, if you're forcing your biceps to work against the resistance of your opposite hand and arm (by pulling your right lower arm toward your shoulder against the resistance of your left hand clasped against the front of your right wrist) be certain at some time during your conditioning routine that you also make the muscles along the *back* of your upper arm (the triceps muscle) do the same amount of work.

When you do a push-up, it's your triceps muscle that strains doing the "pushing-up" maneuver. You can use this exercise to balance any you do with your biceps muscles. All parts of your body have opposing muscles that move your arm, leg, etc. in *opposite* directions. For stomach muscles, your back muscles are their opposing group. Don't neglect them! Use your "weak" side as much as your strong — your left as much as your right side, in other words.

Calisthenics

Calisthenic exercises are the ones that involve *moving* a part or all of your body in one way or another. Walking and jogging are calisthenics. Sit-ups and push-ups also are calisthenics as are swimming and bicycling. Calisthenics develop strength and stamina, and are good heart and lung toners as well.

After you have mastered isometrics, calisthenics can be added slowly to your routine and at your own pace. Remember that it is well to add one calisthenic at a time to your routine until you're adjusted to it.

Weights

The use of the barbell and weights is primarily for development of strength and to increase the size of your muscles. Weights are fine as long as *conservatism* guides your use of them. The standard set of weights comes with a long bar, different sized weights totaling eighty to 100 pounds, flanges and hand grips. There are usually one or two shorter bars for use with one hand and smaller weights as well.

Successful weight lifting is a matter of balance and timing. You would do well to start with only twenty-five or thirty pounds of weights on the long bar. Be certain they are in balance (that the weights are tightened to the bar the same distance from both ends) before using them. Don't overdo with weights. Start slowly and lightly and *gradually work up over a period of months.*

An appendix at the end of this book will show you how to do other important exercises.

You can easily make up your own conditioning routines that are built up, for instance, on the muscle groups that need it the most. The following occupational categories will help you decide where you need help and how to start your program:

Executive

People who work in the general field of business — behind a desk most of the time — fall into this conditioning niche.

The executive usually has poor conditioning in all his muscles, but especially in the abdomen, legs and chest.

Carl is a businessman I know who exemplified this flabby group. Carl could not look down and observe his feet, so great was his abdominal protrusion. Carl enjoyed hunting but his legs would play out after an hour or two in the field. His chest was sunken and his back curved outwardly from chronic dystonia of his chest and upper back muscles. I started Carl out with two calisthenic conditioners because his lungs were in poor shape from too much smoking and he was in serious danger of developing cardiac trouble as are most middle-aged business-men who are out of shape.

Carl profited from jogging and from cycling. The latter served the dual purpose of adding strength and stamina to his weak legs. He started jogging (a slow steady run) just down to the end of his block and back once a day. If he got tired before he reached home again, I instructed him to slow to a walk immediately. It's easy, remember, to stop short of over-exerting yourself. All you need to do is pay attention to what your body tries to tell you. In Carl's case his lungs (uncomfortable breathing) and his heart rate (pounding) were his warning signals. In four weeks, Carl found he could double this jogging distance. He's increased the distance over the months so now he can and does jog a mile a day at least, sometimes twice a day. His "wind" has returned and he can now enjoy hunting and can keep up with any twenty year old.

Carl has learned to use his son's bicycle to run errands and to cover distances he used to do in his car. He and his wife have discovered cycling is a wonderful family diversion, and they go on cycle trips often in the warmer months. In winter, Carl (and his wife) have taken up skiing when cycling is no longer possible. Carl couldn't possibly have considered skiing before his conditioning routine put him in the excellent shape skiing demands.

Manual Labor

People who do manual labor — light, moderate or heavy — do have conditioning problems. Sometimes worse than executives!

Such a man was Joe, a patient I knew who worked in a

foundry. Joe had exceptionally well-developed arms and chest muscles from the heavy weights his job obliged him to handle. Joe also had a pot belly and a chronically unstable back. Not only were these "weak" groups of muscles hardly ever used on his job, his weight carrying often caused him to strain his back.

Joe was placed first on back isometrics. "The "rocking horse" exercise that Jim used previously in this section was the first, and the routine laying flat on the floor on his stomach and using his hip muscles (buttocks) to alternately lift his legs up off the floor was another. Joe could easily do sit-ups for his stomach and so I started him on thirty a day progressing to fifty then seventy-five spread over two sessions a day. Using this routine, Joe eventually lost his pot and can now see both feet when he looks down. His wife had to take in all his pants to accomodate the six inches Joe lost from his waist! And he hasn't had one claim of back strain since starting his conditioning.

Housewife

Rose, a petite housewife whose general muscle tone was good had, nevertheless, a distressing problem: a chronically weak lower back. Rose could work hard all day long in the house with all the washing, cleaning, sweeping and mopping, but what plagued her the most was picking something off the floor or stooping over to clean the tub or pick up the baby. Rose's back responded to a combination of the "leg lift," described previously for Joe at the foundry, and to the "bend-over", a routine done by standing straight, feet about eighteen inches apart, then bending over frontward at the waist until head was hanging between legs such that she could see an object located in back of her such as a lamp on a table. The second move is to bend *backward* at the waist until head extended far enough back to see the same lamp on the table. I instructed Rose to keep her legs perfectly straight at the knees with both bending movements. At first, Rose could do no more than three such bends. After several weeks, she progressed to fifteen and now does twenty a day sometimes, twice a day, to keep her back supple, strong and limber.

Rose has eliminated low back trouble since starting this routine.

Secretary

Female office workers are particularly prone to "spreading fanny," drooping breasts and flabby arms. And like their male counterparts, they are often plagued by pot stomachs. A routine to correct all of these ailments of body framework was perfected by Jane, a thirty-five year old woman who types and files in an office all day long.

On arising, Jane does fifteen or twenty sit-ups. Being a person who enjoys variation, she alternates these with abdominal isometrics as described previously in this section. At still other times, Jane has invented a circular waist twist done with hands on hips and making a complete circle with her torso, bending sharply at each side as well as forward and backward with the motion. Several dozen of these cycles substitute for Jan's sit-ups or isometrics.

She follows these variations with deep knee bends and squat jumps in which she bends at the knees to a squatting position and jumps by thrusting upward with her lower legs four times in one position, then turns a quarter turn to the right and four more jumps and so on until several complete circles are made in this squat jump position. At night, before retiring, Jane does either twenty push-ups (contrary to popular belief, *push-ups are indeed good for females*) or uses a small bar (about twelve inches long) with two and a half pounds of weight on either end for circular motion with the weight held in one hand, arm extended out straight in front and all movement at the shoulder. This combination has tightened her pectoral muscles and keeps Jane's breasts firm, upright and trim.

CONDITIONING BONUSES YOURS FOR THE ASKING

You can tell from the cases in this section that people vary somewhat in their problems of muscle conditioning and vary almost infinitely in what they use to correct them. You can do just as well by using the three basic types of conditioners and fitting them to your particular problem. The point to remember is to be *consistent* — a certain block of time twice daily to be set aside for this important project. Early A.M. and late P.M.

are excellent for isometrics, calisthenics and weights. One common "bonus" among people like those in this section who've found the young life again with conditioning is that every one of them tell me that not only do they get the bargain of youthful figures and pep again, *but that their minds work better, brighter and more efficiently for their efforts!*

This isn't surprising at all. From every nerve cell that stimulates muscle fibers to contract, a pathway exists that ends up in the brain — the seat of your mind! Not only can impulses travel down from brain to muscle in this nerve trunk, but also the reverse: impulses travel from muscle to brain. This reverse flow of toning impulses set up by physical conditioning acts as a mind toning device. The best minds today are found in people who are in top physical condition! Why not take advantage of this tremendous bonus of a better mind by starting your conditioning today? You'll never regret it and you'll have a younger more agile mind for your trouble!

CHAPTER SUMMARY

1. Diet and physical conditioning go hand in hand. Embark on both at once for maximum youth-inducing results.
2. Your framework, bones, connective tissue and muscles, ages with disuse. The easy way to reverse this aging in your body's framework is through regular and continuous conditioning routines done at least twice a day for fifteen to thirty minutes. A small price to pay for healthful vigorous youth-power.
3. The three types of exercises, calisthenics, isometrics and weights, can be used in infinite variation to suit your problems. Innovate! Find different ways to keep *all* your muscles in tone *all* the time!
4. One of the most welcome bonuses from physical toning is that your mind is also toned for more robust inventive and creative thinking. Take advantage of your natural mind stimulator by starting your conditioning routines today!

4

How to Keep Your Mind Young, Incisive and Razor Sharp

Have you noticed how our age of super-specialization seems to be spliting everything up into still smaller parts? How medical specialties are carving up your organism so much that you may have to visit six or eight different doctors for a single ailment? One specialty for some years has attempted to separate mind completely from its attached body and deal with it as though it existed separately — I believe psychiatrists will finally come to the point where they must reunite body with mind.

In this section I'll discuss your most precious possession, your mind. I want you to understand fully how your mind works so that you can begin to tap its youth reserves and discover some of its remarkable potentials.

In your progress toward youth, mind is the driving force — the dynamo from which you derive youthful energy. I want you to learn how to keep this well-oiled dynamo functioning smoothly all the time. I want you to understand how to train your mind to aid you in several areas of youth building; how to focus the power of your mind on any task at hand so you can multiply your efficiency ten-fold. One of today's greatest tragedies is the fading away of one's mind. I want to show you how to prevent this untimely fade-out, and how to keep it as trim at seventy as it was at seventeen.

MENTAL TONE MEANS YOUTH RESERVE

Your mind is a good deal like muscle — to function efficiently, it must *be used.* The more use it gets, the better your mind does for you. Unlike muscle, however, you need never fear *overusing* it. It can't get "muscle-bound" from too much use! It *can* get weak and out of phase from underuse!

The wonderful thing about your mind is that if it's become sluggish and rusty, *the potential is still there to bring it back —* to restore its fantastic power again.

Nerves are direct extensions of your mind. They penetrate and control virtually every organ, muscle, blood vessel and gland in your body. For this reason, you have at your command the means to bring into sharp focus *total body control* through mind!

And how do you promote mental tone? Easy. You challenge your mind! You present it problems, offer it goals and make it overcome obstacles. And you learn. Mental conditioning restores tone to your mind just as physical conditioning restores muscles. With better mental tone comes, among other things, better physical conditioning, and better physical conditioning, remember, tones up mind. You can't lose!

HOW TO PUT YOUR MIND
TO WORK FOR YOUTHFULNESS

Concentration

Strangely enough, your mind does some of its most astonishing work quite unbeknownst to you. It does this in the so-called *subconscious* area — the area that lies outside the day-to-day reality when you're awake and grinding away at whatever routine you're a part of. Your mind's *conscious* area takes care of making you *aware* of what's going on around you and goes about the business of putting into effect the material delivered to it from subconscious. You can start right now to influence your subconscious mind to begin youth building.

Having some difficulty with the diet routine outlined in the second chapter? Think you need drugs to control that appetite? Nonsense! Start controlling hunger pangs with your subconscious mind.

Here's what to do:

Just before you're ready to drift off to sleep tonight, concentrate on just one thing for about three minutes: That you'll go through the next day without hunger pangs. Repeat this challenge again and again, allowing nothing else to cloud your thoughts. Just this one challenge regarding appetite control. *Then put the subject out of your thinking completely.* Forget it! Go to sleep. You'll be surprised to find your pangs have materially lessened the next day. Do it again the next night and the next. Soon, complete appetite control will be yours!

To reinforce the challenge, do the same concentrating sometime during the day. Relax completely, close your eyes and repeat the phrase, "My stomach will remain perfectly comfortable until the next meal (or snack)." *Then forget it —* submerge the challenge completely from your conscious thinking. You'll be amazed. It will work like a charm!

This is concentration using autosuggestion, the same technique a hypnotist uses on his subject when he is "under hypnosis." The difference is that you're not handing your will over to someone else — *you're in control at all times.*

HOW ROGER USED MIND OVER MATTER

A patient named Roger had just such a problem. When I first put Roger on a diet designed according to the plan given in Chapter 2, he argued that he'd been through all this before. "Won't work," he said. "I've tried 'em all and I know I'll have to have drugs to control my appetite," he added. Roger was a forty year old five foot-ten incher who weighed 196 pounds. About forty pounds too much! I did convince him to try, and to talk to me again in about two weeks to see how things were coming. Two weeks later, he appeared in the office with a smirk on his face. I knew what he was going to say. He said he couldn't hack the hunger pangs and would I please give him a prescription for appetite control.

When I said there was yet another alternative, he looked at me like he thought I was balmy. "Look," I said. "You've always prided yourself on your 'iron will.' You've boasted there wasn't anything you couldn't do if you set your mind on it, right?" He nodded affirmatively. He couldn't do otherwise, because he'd made such a boast when we were discussing his physical conditioning a few weeks before.

It turned out that Roger's appetite problem was at dinner time and again at bedtime following his toning regime. Roger was an employee of an industrial concern and often met clients at lunch where the ritual of putting away two or three martinis before lunch and then enough food for two people was the rule. I convinced him to forego the martinis and to eat only a light lunch with a mid-afternoon snack. This controlled his blood sugar cycle so he didn't have quite the voracious appetite at dinner time. Then I convinced him to set aside just five or ten minutes after lunch in a quiet place where he could stretch out and really relax, and to concentrate on the challenge that he would not have hunger pangs during the entire afternoon. He was instructed to repeat the challenge immediately following dinner.

Roger pooh-poohed the idea and told me he thought it sounded like a lot of hocus-pocus to him. Then I asked him where he thought his "iron will" came from — what it was that produced all this determination. He pondered the question a bit then smiled. "You know," he said, "I never looked at it that way before. "I produce it inside." It worked. Within a week, Roger had control of his appetite and kept it controlled during the seven months it took him to get down to ideal weight. He's never strayed from it since.

Yes, you can exert mind over matter! And a good place to start is with your body. Plan to start today.

The Role of Will Power

You've met strong-willed persons, I'm sure. Where do they get it? Where does that disciplined, unwavering will come from? From the subconscious mind, as a matter of fact. When I talked about a hypnotized person a bit ago, recall I said that conscious mind "stands aside" temporarily and that subconscious mind is laid bare. But the most expert hypnotist will tell you that they can't give you any commands or orders that are against your basic will — against your natural grain, in other words. This is because your subconscious mind holds in it all those things that over the years have gone into the making of your personality — the essence of *you,* which is your will. Can this be influenced, be stimulated to bigger and better things? You bet it can! And this very "influenceability" of will is what makes your mind young, healthy and strong! Having some trouble, for example, with your physical conditioning routine? Can't really get it off the ground? Or persist at it?

Try this:

> In bed tonight, just before you doze off to sleep, repeat this phrase for about two or three minutes over and over, allowing nothing else to enter your thinking: "I *will awaken* tomorrow ready, willing and eager to exercise. I will *want* to exercise again before I go to bed tomorrow night." In a short time, perhaps a week or so, you'll be pleasantly surprised at how much your will has been influenced. How much you seem to desire all of a sudden to really want to go through with the routine, and how uncomfortable you'll feel if you don't!

HOW WILL POWER TURNED THE
YOUTH TONING SWITCH ON FOR LANA

Women, especially, have to be "sold" on physical conditioning. I can't blame them — often their daily chores involve what they consider God's plenty in the way of exercise, what with the housework, grocery shopping and so on. But women do need it. Often more than men.

I recall having a difficult time making a patient named Lana see this point. And it was especially important for her because she had about sixty-eight pounds to trim off. Diet alone would do it for Lana, but because of her particular build — large bust and protuberant abdomen — she would have loose skin and flabby muscles hanging from her figure like draperies if she didn't get into a solid physical conditioning routine along with dieting.

Lana, like Roger, stuck to the idea that drugs to control her appetite were all she needed. "After all," she said, "I've done it before. And those pills really made me go!" She was right, in a way. She had done it before, but she gained all the weight back in a few months. And the pills really did "make her go." But she forgot to add that they made her nervous as a wet hen in the process, and when it came time to stop the drug, she found it very difficult to do so.

I managed to convince Lana that it lay within herself to accomplish the goal of physical toning. I asked her to set her alarm clock twenty minutes ealier than usual to awaken in the morning. Then I asked her to repeat the following challenge in bed at night just before dozing off to sleep: "I will awaken at 6:25 in the morning." At the same time she was repeating this phrase, I instructed her to visualize the face of a clock with the hands pointing at 6:25 (she usually got up at 6:45). I told Lana I wanted her completely weaned from the alarm. And when she arose, I wanted her to do her morning physical work-out before she started one other thing.

It took Lana only five days to master her "mental alarm." She awoke amazingly close to 6:25 whenever she "willed" it, and after two weeks of exercising told me that she felt many times the woman she used to be because of the physical routine "stirred her up" mentally and she literally whipped through the day, with energy to spare.

Later, I had Lana do the same thing with her evening toning routine. I asked her to lay down on a couch or bed and concentrate on wanting to exercise before retiring at night. It worked! In four weeks, Lana told me she actually felt "letdown" if she missed either one of her two physical toning routines! Lana lost her sixty-eight pounds in about eleven months. Today she looks about fifteen years younger for the effort and hasn't a fold of skin or one sagging muscle hanging on her body — she has recaptured a lost youth!

PROBLEM SOLVING MADE EASY

Ever had the provoking experience of going to bed with an unsolved problem on your mind? If so, you didn't get much sleep. Sometimes you spend days, even weeks, with the problem "on your mind" without its getting worked out. It's so easy to use those dormant areas in your subconscious mind to solve problems! Next time you have a perplexing problem on your hands, try the following:

> When you retire and just before you're ready to doze off, concentrate. Concentrate on the problem and repeat for two or three minutes over and over, "I will awaken with the answer to . . . " (whatever the problem is). Let nothing else enter your mind. Then, forget about the problem en-

tirely — challenge your subconscious mind and submerge your problem into the subconscious by putting it out of your conscious thinking completely.

One of three things will happen. You may well awaken later that night out of a sound sleep or the next morning with the answer standing out in your mind as though someone just printed it out for you! You may suddenly get the answer the next day right in the middle of something you're doing that hasn't the remotest connection with your problem. It will "flash" like a neon sign. Or it may take several nights of deep concentration in the manner I described, depending on how practiced you are at concentrating. But the solution will come, be absolutely assured! And the depth or complexity of the problem won't make a whit of difference. Your mind will crank out the answer (or answers) if you challenge it to.

HOW CLIFF USED HIS SUBCONSCIOUS POWER

A man I know named Cliff is a good example of someone who has learned just how valuable an asset his mind really is. Cliff is a senior executive in retail manufacturing. While working with Cliff on a weight and physical conditioning problem one time, I'd mentioned to him about using his subconscious dormant areas to help. Casually, I'd also mention how mind can solve health problems if challenged to do so.

Cliff decided, without telling me at the time, to put the statement to the acid test. It seems Cliff had a tough complicated problem with product distribution. He'd labored days over the thing which had appeared suddenly in his expanding business and soon became a crisis. The president was on Cliff's neck to get cracking; the vice president was chewing on Cliff about every day and the branch offices were screaming for answers. Cliff was developing heart burn, indigestion and insomnia from wrestling with his problem all of which had him aging rapidly. Then he tried the challenge I flung to him.

Later, Cliff told me it took only thirty-six hours from the night of the first concentration and challenge to come up with an answer that involved utilizing a newly formed computer service: Special telephone hookups in all his offices and a new method of warehouse inventory which Cliff's mind "threw in" as a bonus!

Cliff became a believer. He uses this method routinely for all such issues, and he gets results. So firm is his belief in the system and so adept has he become in using it, he tells me he keeps pad and pen on the nightstand by his bed because he often awakes three or four hours following the challenge with the answer coming through in his mind like a tape recording. He jots the points down and resumes a restful relaxing sleep!

Cliff also swears that using the method has seemed to pull him out of what he'd looked on as a thinking rut. He told me sometime later that his mind works smoother, faster and more efficiently during the day and that decisions he used to put off for days, he now makes in a few minutes. And they're invariably the right ones!

Why not cash in on Cliff's experience? Learn to use your mind for the hundreds of problems that plague you and age you before your time.

FAMILY CATASTROPHE AVOIDED BY USING MIND

Mary's case is representative of what must be tens of thousands that happen to people every year. She used her mind to help solve a most difficult situation, and she freely declares that without this powerful tool she might well be destitute today!

Mary had an alcoholic husband and two teen-aged youngsters who were beginning a life of juvenile delinquency. Both of them had two minor scrapes with police authorities and were headed for more. The trouble with her husband's alcohol problem was that he steadfastly denied there was a problem and continued to booze it up every chance he got. He was also beginning to carouse with other women. Mary was hysterical with worry and became haggard in appearance. She was nervous as a cat and begged for tranquillizers to help steady her frayed nerves. I had a long chat with Mary and told her that at least some of the solution to her troubles lay in her own mind, and that she would do well to try helping things before her situation went from bad to worse.

Reluctantly, and only after I prescribed a mild tranqualizer for the next few nights, Mary said she would try. The effect was enormous! Normally a rather shy person, Mary went to her husband's boss that same week and explained the situation.

He was sympathetic. He called Mary's husband into his office the next day and really laid it on the line, in accordance with Mary's plan. He told him to find help for his drinking problem or he'd discharge him — no questions asked, no quarter given. The husband joined Alcoholics Anonymous and has been on the wagon since. Next, Mary called a family conference — husband and both children. She, likewise, laid it on the line. She "dressed down" the children and told her husband she held him directly responsible for them if they didn't shape up. All present realized Mary meant business. Father, now faced with loss of job, discovered his carousing days were over when Mary said in no uncertain terms that if this foolishness didn't come to an immediate and permanent halt, she'd hire a lawyer and sue him for separate maintenance, and turn the children over to juvenile court for prosecution if they didn't shape up!

The treatment sounds rough, but this was the way the solution came through after a few nights of subconscious challenge. She followed through. Today, Mary is happy, the children are on the straight and narrow and are doing well in school, and Mary's husband is an ideal father and husband.

I've often wondered since watching Mary's story unfold, how many domestic crises might be avoided in this country if just one of the partners involved learned to use the power residing in his own mind!

BONUSES FROM MIND POWER

Someone asked me just recently whether I put any credence in ESP, (extra-sensory perception). I replied that not only did I put credence in it, but I'm firmly convinced that this field is one of the most overlooked areas in scientific research today!

Telepathy

You and I and everybody have an extra something in our minds that enables us to communicate with other than our five senses. This "sixth sense" is telepathy. I'm convinced of this, and I'm convinced that anyone who tries can develop his sixth sense to a considerable degree. I've explained how this can be done in an appendix at the end of the book.

Clairvoyance

The ability to perceive things that occur at distances is not at all new or unusual. Documented cases exist in profusion. The ability of some people to "know" something that happened in the past or that will happen in future is likewise documented. Both these faculties I believe are also part of the human mind. They can be developed with practice.

Psychokinesis

We have already seen an instance of mind over matter in the case history of Roger, discussed earlier in this section. There are many others. For example, when you teach your child that two plus two is four, and he believes and accepts this as fact, you have, indeed, influenced matter (his brain) with your mind. The extension of mind over inanimate objects is a fascinating field likewise lacking in good scientific research. It lies waiting today as a new frontier. I have hopes that the whole field of ESP will soon be explored by scientists so that we all may learn how to fully utilize ESP to stay younger.

KEEPING MIND YOUNG

The secret of preventing your mind from aging is quite simple: Keep it active! Perceptive to new ideas! This includes the following:

1. No matter who you are or what you do, develop and cultivate the habit of tackling a subject completely outside your field of work — something that's always interested you — and become an authority on it. Read, study, learn, take courses (most colleges and universities offer non-credit courses in the evenings in virtually every subject) and pick brains. Then, contribute. Ask yourself questions about the subject that seem to you unanswered — be a nit-picker — speak out — get *involved* in it.

2. Purposely take on problems and situations that you've always avoided because they seem "too complicated" or too tough to handle. Stay with it until you work completely through it. Even if it takes years!

3. Plan now the things you're going to get involved with when retirement comes along. Outline a course of study for yourself. Set goals and don't stop until they are realized! If anything, get more involved when you retire than you are right now!
4. Look up the resources in your area. Public libraries offer films, tapes, books, old manuscripts and lectures. Don't let this invaluable reservoir of knowledge go to waste!
5. Remember, the secret of youthful mind is to keep it busy!

CHAPTER SUMMARY

1. The vital essence of youth is the body-mind, mind-body influence. The better physical tone you're in, the better the tone of your mind, and vice versa.
2. Restore your mind to better youthful efficiency by challenging your dormant subconscious areas to more and better achievements. The keys for this challenge are concentration and will power.
3. The most valuable asset you have for steady youth is your mind. Use it to solve your perplexing problems and to expand your mental capacity.
4. Keep a youthful mind by keeping it fully and continuously active.

5

How to Control Your
Inner Organism Cycles
for More Lasting
Youthful Energy

Did you know your body is governed by a series of cycles?
That virtually all your organs, glands and tissues are subject to
these repeating periods of activity and inactivity?

You will learn more about these cycles and how to control
them in this chapter. You will learn how to utilize your cycles
to stay younger and live longer, healthier lives.

Just as the huge galaxy of which our solar system is only a
speck is subject to cycles, so does every part of your body
respond to natural rhythms or cycles. Knowing what they are,
how they operate and how to control them will further aid you
in looking and feeling younger all the time.

There are many things you do every day — patterns of habit
you succumb to — that work as anti-cycles and add years of
unnecessary wear and tear to your organism. You'll learn about
such anti-cycles and how to neutralize them. You can take
advantage of weather and seasonal cycles as well and learn
to properly fuse them with those of your organism to gain
years of sparkling and youthful health.

HOW TO CONTROL YOUR ORGANIC CYCLES

You can learn from Van's case a lesson in body-mind cycles.
Van is a young man with a good job and lots of potential,
but he never gets ahead, as he put it to me one day. Never
seems to make the grade with his bosses. "I can't seem to pull
anything off the way I plan it," was the way he stated the case.
When I began to quiz him about why it was that nothing ever
seemed to go right, he heaved a great sigh like a condemned
man might, and gave me the details. Seems Van spent late

hours at night working out details of his sales operation. He got little sleep and even that was fretful. The next morning he was loggy and listless. He gulped down much black coffee, ate very little, if any, breakfast and dashed off to work. But by the time he reached his office, his energy was gone and his ideas, worked out so carefully the night before, seemed to disintegrate and appear worthless.

"Everything comes apart at the seams," he said, bitterly.

Van's is a common problem. He's reversed his natural mind-body cycle — he should be arranging his sales schedule in the morning when he first arises, when his mind is at its clearest and sharpest. He should have a good *relaxing* night's sleep for as many hours as his organism normally requires. In fact, when he started this simple routine he began to make head-way at work — his sales increased, the deals went through and his bosses noticed it! Van took advantage of before-bed exercises to help him relax. He lost weight and his muscles took on tone again. He looked ten and felt twenty years younger in three months' time. You can take advantage of Van's youthful change — start today to put *your* body-mind cycle in phase!

Bone, Muscle and Nerve Cycles

Your bones are made of protein with calcium salts impregnated on them for hardness. This calcium is on the move — back and forth from bones to blood stream all the time. When your muscles are made to pull extra-hard on their bony attachments the calcium is prompted to go to the bones to strengthen them. Your skeleton becomes stronger and more resistant to stresses and strains. Van, in the case mentioned a bit ago, further aided his own cause by his exercise routine. The result was a better controlled calcium cycle and a younger bony skeleton as a result!

Muscles, too, have their cycles. The health of a muscle cell depends on the back and forth movement of certain minerals from the inside to the outside of its walls. This is the muscle mineral cycle. Sodium, potassium and calcium are three key minerals in this vital cycle. When calcium moves from muscle to bone in response to exercise, muscle cells become more active and able to respond more quickly. Coordination is increased. Too much calcium makes muscles listless, unresponsive and weak. How do you control this cycle? Simple: Van did it when he began to lose weight and exercise. When he adjusted his diet so that skim milk and plenty of fruit became a regular part of his diet, all the sodium and potassium he needed were supplied in ample amounts. So, get with a more youthful body today through control of your mineral cycles!

Van's case illustrates yet another cycle he'd let get out of adjustment — the nerve cycle. When the day is ended, nerves, including the thirteen billion that make up your brain, need to be rejuvenated. Van, by stewing and fretting with his work half the night and by frittering away precious relaxing sleep the other half threw his nerve cycle completely out of phase. If nerves don't get a chance to recover after a day's work, they begin to age prematurely. You need quiet, relaxing nightmare-free sleep every night to control your nerve cycle and keep those nerve cells young! Whether you're used to two or twelve hours of sleep at night, get that much to prevent aging nerves.

Gland and Organ Cycles

Recall our discussion of the endocrine glands — those vital chemical factories that make the hormones that control your entire body chemistry. The pituitary master gland, small as it is, regulates all the rest of your endocrine cycles.

You readers who are women will hardly need reminding or tutoring about the menstrual cycle. This regularly occurring three or four weekly cycle is the basis for human reproduction. Not long ago, I talked with a charming lady I'll call Nancy. Nancy was a journalist for a local newspaper and did a lot of writing in her capacity as Woman's Page Editor. She told me that about once or twice a month, she became stale — unable to crank out her usually vital and interesting comments on the fashions of the day and so on. "I don't know, maybe its just old-age," she said wistfully. She was forty-five years old, but certainly didn't look it. I told her I found that hard to believe and questioned her about what else was going on during these "stale" periods. It soon came out that they were always just before her menstrual cycle. She was approaching menopause, and having less active periods though a little more often than she did, say, five or ten years ago. She also felt depressed and a little jittery. Two cycles were out of adjustment here. I'll go into the second of these a bit later.

Nancy's is a common story. The female hormone (estrogen) level, high and sustained during the greater part of the menstrual cycle, takes a sudden dip just before menstrual bleeding occurs. With this dip comes tenseness, jitters and "blue" moods. Of course, Nancy couldn't be productive in her writing during these brief periods. Her organic cycle wasn't up to being productive or creative. Nancy soon learned to turn her attention to duties that involved less creative output and more routine chores at her newspaper. She soon discovered that she didn't have to go through the frustration of poor production during these times of the month. She let her menstrual cycle run its course and then got back on the production track when it was over. She will soon stop menstruating altogether and may look to an end to these sticky cycles.

Importance of Blood Sugar Cycle

A man I'll call Chuck was stuck with yet another organic cycle let-down. He was very like Van whom we've talked about. Chuck was hard-driving, on the way up, but vastly overweight and flabby. His chief complaint was grogginess, inability to concentrate, nervousness during the day and increasing intolerance of his family. In talking to Chuck, I learned that it was his habit to eat nothing for breakfast, to drink six to eight cups of coffee in the morning and to gorge himself with a large lunch loaded with carbohydrate at noon, often with a martini or two if at a business luncheon. After a gruelling day at work, he'd come home, down three or four "slugs" of gin or whiskey. From this point on, he was, as he put it, "shot for the evening." Small wonder! Chuck was out of phase with one of the most fundamental of his organic cycles, his blood sugar cycle. Let's take a look at what happened to this cycle in Chuck's case.

1. No breakfast; three times too much black coffee; blood sugar driven down to extremely low levels.
2. Loaded up with too much carbohydrate (starchy) foods and excessive alcohol; pancreas stimulated to pour out

three times too much insulin; sugar burned away; too much insulin produces nervousness, irritability and stimulates liver to pour out reserves of sugar which also burned up.

3. Rush home to more alcohol; sugar levels driven down even further; lethargy, grouchiness, even stupor results.

You can't cheat on your blood sugar cycle! Besides oxygen, the other necessary ingredient for all body cells in high quantity and at all times is an adequate sugar level. Deprive brain cells, for example, of sugar to burn in ample amounts as energy for just three minutes and you have destruction of brain cells! Chuck recovered from his disrupted sugar cycle by following the basic premises necessary to prevent the low blood sugar levels:

1. Weight at minimum levels for height-age and frame. (See tables at end of book.)
2. Muscles firmly and constantly exercised and toned.
3. Alcohol intake cut 80 percent and taken only after arriving home before dinner or at bedtime *after* exercise routine.
4. Black coffee drinking cut 90 percent. Skim milk or carbohydrates taken with it so blood sugar will not be driven down.
5. Meal habits revised: four to six smaller meals eaten during the day instead of two huge ones. Protein 65 percent; Carbohydrate 25 percent, and fat 10 percent of total eaten.

Result: In three months, total control of blood sugar cycle and fifteen to twenty years added to healthful life span!

You can have just as good results as Chuck did by following the simple low blood sugar rules. Start today to add years to your life!

TAKING THE MYSTERY
OUT OF YOUR SEX CYCLE

Much has been said and written about sex cycles. Most of it is fictional. In the past twenty years we've learned much about human sexual behavior thanks to the painstaking work of such people as Kinsey and his associates and to the radical departure from the usual methods of investigation of such people as Masters and Johnson.

Basically, human sexual urge is governed by arousal through a member of the opposite sex. Many things go into arousal: the situation, the setting and so on. On a broad scale, sexual urge is seen to be subject to cycles.

Women

The female's sex cycles are closely controlled by her menstrual cycles. After menopause, this cycle is smoothed out and gives way to the same long-term cycles that govern the male sex cycle. Recall the blue moods of Nancy I talked about earlier in this section. Part of this blue mood was brought on by frustration of her sexual cycle. The sex urge in women seems highest in the last part of the cycle — and appears to reach a crest just before menstruation begins. When Nancy, a happily married woman, began to give vent to this urge, her frustration lessened and her moodiness showed improvement almost immediately.

Men

The cycles of sex among men are not so clear-cut as with women. That the male sex urge waxes and wanes in rather long-term cycles is clear. The facts that govern these long-term cycles aren't clear. Many things are known that do interfere with a man's sexual urge. Among the most important of these are:

1. Being overweight.
2. Too much alcohol indulgence.
3. Too little or too much attention to muscular development.
4. A host of drugs taken for a variety of conditions.

Both Van and Chuck whose problems I've discussed were also plagued with diminished sexual urges. When they began to control their organic cycles, their sexual cycles also fell into line. It's plain to see that in following their improvement plan, they both eliminated the first three factors in the preceding list of sexually retarding situations. Neither had a drug problem, but there are thousands who do.

Today, the most common offending drug that inhibits the sexual urge in men are the tranquilizers. No one knows how many millions of these pills are taken in this country. The problem is so common that I routinely ask men with marital difficulties whether they are taking such drugs. If they are, they will be relatively impotent sexually as long as they keep taking them.

I recently talked with a man in his mid-thirties who had been taking potent tranquillizers for five years for a serious mental problem. He hadn't had normal sexual relations with his wife for three years! This case makes one wonder about the long range effects of the so-called wonder drugs of today. Are we really doing people a favor in such a situation? Certainly, this man has his mental problem under much better control than before. But his marital situation is beginning to deteriorate. His wife is talking of divorce.

This man's drug therapy is being reduced. If it could be stopped, his potency would return — and so would his psychosis. You may see now what I meant by *preventive* mental illness in the preceding section. The only good answer to today's mental health problem is *prevention*. And prevention is absolutely hinged on the considerations of a young mind — on learning how to head off trouble before it begins to age you prematurely!

HOW TO GAIN CONTROL OF YOUR ENVIRONMENT CYCLES

Ever stop to think about all the things you live with day in and day out that add years prematurely to your organism? The simplest thing to do to discover this for yourself is to take a few minutes and jot down a list of all the things that cause you to get frustrated, angry and put you into a rut. You'll be surprised to find how many of these "life's little aggravations" occur in cycles that you can exert control over — and live longer youthfully as a result.

Family

I know a family who gained control over its "family cycles" by analyzing why things didn't seem ever to go right with its members. Among others, this group consisting of Mom, Dad, two daughters and a son who constantly stewed, fretted and got into knock-down, drag-out squabbles. When they began to take a look at some of their cycles, the reason for the strife became clear.

For one thing, this family failed to account for the "school cycle" — the children, all in junior and senior high, went to school nine months of the year, then had three months off in the summer. No plans were ever made regarding what occupied their time during those three months. The oldest daughter had a tough time finding part-time work and the younger two weren't of hirable age yet. The kids were bored; Mom and Dad were unconcerned. The two younger kids soon found themselves in trouble. The son was caught running with some others his age shooting holes in neighbors' windows with bee-bee guns. The daughter was discovered swimming in the nude at a nearby lake in mixed company.

When the family learned to cope with this free-time cycle, their troubles largely disappeared. Both Dad and Mom spent a good deal more time with their children during the summer. Instead of each family member kind of going off in his own little world, the family took vacations *together* and saw to it that each member got to do something on the trip that interested *him.* They learned to do things as a family rather than just "to each his own." The parents began to watch their children more closely during the busy school year and to take a genuine interest in what was going on rather than to use the school term as "a break for Mom and Dad and the worries of the summer."

In doing this, Mom and Dad also became acutely aware of their children's cycles — children also have sexual and other organism cycles that have to be dealt with. They learned how to channel these restless and frustrating cycles into productivity — to keep the children busy with projects that syphoned off their excess energy into paths that kept them out of trouble. With three women menstruating in this household, everyone eventually learned not to raise thorny problems during these times and learned to tolerate better the emotion-filled premenstrual periods that previously sent the family into cycles of bickering and frustration.

Work

Probably no one will ever truly appreciate all the "guff" or torment a breadwinner must swallow at his daily chore. Everybody has a threshold for guff. When it's surpassed, something's got to give. At this point, the pent-up guff, real or imagined, explodes either inside or outside. When it goes inside, it knaws at the intestines, the stomach, the blood pressure and so on. It often gets released at home where the unfortunate victims may not even know what caused Dad's "stack blowing."

In a recent survey conducted among workers in various fields, it was clearly shown that such "work cycles" depended on three main circumstances: the health of the business, the health of the boss and the health of the worker himself. If the state of health of any of these three areas was poor, so also were working conditions. And what did the people interviewed say they did to cope with these cycles? Three in four depended on channeling methods and the fourth preferred to go directly to the source of the "trouble" and "have it out" with the individuals involved.

This points out something I've been trying to get across thus far with staying younger and feeling younger: that it's during the very times of excess stresses and strains that you need to pay even more special attention to what you're doing to your organism.

For channeling in response to such cycles in your business, whatever it may be, you might be interested in knowing that in one instance during the interview mentioned previously, an executive did it by swimming four times the length of the swimming pool at his club during the noon hour. Another, a woman who worked part time in a large department store, did her channeling by immersing herself in sewing and knitting, two hobbies she liked and enjoyed.

Another man said he made it a point to double his efforts during these cycles — he was in selling and he doubled his calls and sales. He said this wore him physically but he'd learned from experience that he weathered the cycle storms much better even so.

Since you have now mastered physical conditioning and mental concentration as a part of staying, looking and feeling young, you have at your fingertips one or more excellent ways of channeling in response to your work cycles. Make use of what you've learned to live longer and stay younger on the job!

Weather

That weather affects the human organism has long been known. How it does this and to what exact extent is a field in itself and has barely been scratched. Next time a low pressure system with a storm approaches your area, observe small children. You'll notice they're more excitable, more aggressive and "brattish" and more difficult to control than at other times. Even the flying insects bite more often and harder during the periods of approaching storms. Factories and mental institutions have reported diminished production and efficiency and increased episodes of phychosis, respectively, during low pressure systems and approaching storms, all other considerations being equal.

In general, most people notice they're more efficient and productive during periods of changes in weather patterns such as occur in the fall and spring seasons of the year. These two seasons are also noted for their increased incidence of ulcers and nervous disorders.

For some time it's been known that people perform better, think more clearly and are most rational when the air they're breathing contains a higher number of negatively charged particles than positively charged particles.

You might profit from the following rules of thumb regarding weather and your efficiency:

1. Put off important decisions and tackling tough problems in the face of an approaching storm and a low pressure system.
2. Plan some physical activity for groups of kids in the face of a falling barometer. Don't expect them to be content or to be models of deportment with tasks requiring mental concentration.

3. Put those important plans of action and those ideas you've been mulling over into high gear in the spring and fall of the year if you can. Your chances of success are higher and your ability to carry through is greater. Don't try to be creative during a low pressure storm!

As to other cycles that are well known around us, and how they affect our performance, our thinking and our actions, much study yet remains to be done. For example, huge sunspots occur on our sun in cycles. These vast areas of solar flare cause tremendous energies in the form of radiation to be released and strike our planet's atmosphere in fantastic quantities. It's known that such radiation affects the performance of radio and TV and that it causes other effects such as the aurora borealis (colored lights) in our polar regions. Do these cycles of the sun also affect our health? Do they alter our thinking? Do they cause long range changes in plant and animal life? They probably do. But exactly how, no one can say at present.

Perhaps our entire universe is in the midst of a great cycle. At least one expert in the field of astrophysics believes that the universe first began as a blowing apart of all the solid matter now contained in it, and that, in time, when the blown-apart matter reaches a certain distance, it will reverse its direction and again eventually condense into a solid "ball" of matter, the cycle repeating itself infinitely.

Be this as it may, your aging process can be slowed if you begin to recognize cycles and with their control, affect your well-being.

AVOIDING THE ANTI-YOUTH CYCLES THAT
SPEED UP YOUR AGING PROCESS

I'd like to point out to you six anti-youth cycles and show you how you can avoid them. These anti-youth cycles affect both organic and environmental cycles and with their control, your aging process will slow up. They are:

1. The drudgery anti-cycle.
2. The aging body anti-cycle.

3. The fallow mind anti-cycle.
4. The low blood sugar anti-cycle.
5. The sludge anti-cycle.
6. The disease anti-cycle.

Drudgery

If you can avoid getting into ruts, you can avoid needless aging. Ruts with their attending drudgery add years to what can be a comfortable life. Why does drudgery add years? Because drudgery takes you out of the mainstream of vital living and puts your mind and body into a state of rapid deterioration from disuse.

Van, Chuck, and Nancy, the cases I discussed earlier in this section, all showed unmistakable signs of drudgery and rut-trodding. When they took steps to lift themselves out of their respective pigeon-holes, they proceeded to look and feel younger. They were, in fact, younger people for their effort.

I talked with a man recently who holds a responsible position with a large corporation. This man told me that every four or five years (he's been with the company for twenty-three years) he requests a change of jobs from his bosses and he gets it. He goes into a completely different phase of his company's vast operations, starts in not necessarily at the bottom because he's at least familiar with the company's other departments, but in new environs. Change has become a challenge for this man. And he's profited greatly. The man hasn't had a sick day in the twenty years I've known him. He stays alert, bright and on the go in spite of the fact he's past the usual retirement age of sixty-five years. His company has made an exception to its general policy of retirement because of the very fact that he's more useful to them now than any five or six new younger men. I think we all have a lot to learn from this experience which is, by the way, not unique with this man but represents, I believe, a sign of the changing times. I sincerely hope so, at least. I believe the main reason for this man's present fit mental and physical condition and, more importantly, his *usefulness* to the company he works for (not to mention to him self) is the fact that he took deliberate steps years ago to avoid drudgery.

Aging Body

An organism that's allowed to degenerate and deteriorate is useless. I say allowed, because that's generally what happens — people simply let the ravages of age overtake them and do nothing to stop it. I have seen dozens of elderly people — people beyond the age of seventy-five — literally raised from the dead simply by dint of someone's caring enough to get them up and out of their beds, and involved in some kind of physical activity.

In the first four sections of this book you've been introduced to people who have stopped their aging processes by instilling youthful vigor into aging bodies through attention to diet and exercise. Many times, mastery of section IV dealing with mind control is a necessary pre-requisite to get your body into shape. You can retard aging by getting your body young again — start it today!

Fallow Mind

I've yet to meet anyone who kept his mind active that didn't remain young mentally. The modern tendency, of course, is let the mind go fallow once the working years are ended. This is probably the worst mistake you will ever make.

An oil company executive retired at age sixty-five. He'd never had a sick day in his life until he stopped doing what he'd always done — trouble shooting all over the world for his company. He developed arthritis, an intestinal disorder and an extremely nasty disposition shortly after he "let up." When this man became actively involved in something again, all his afflictions improved and he became a new person. His hobby had always been tinkering with watches. He began to construct, repair and remodel watches and clocks for his friends. Soon, he developed a business and went 'back to work' after retirement. He regained his youth! So can you if you take steps now to get that mind of yours back to work.

Low Blood Sugar

If you supply vital sugar to your trillions of body cells and keep your levels of sugar at optimum peaks, aging will be slowed down immeasurably. Chuck, the man I discussed earlier in this section, did this by following just five basic rules. For a more elaborate discussion of how to keep your blood sugar at optimum levels for a healthy and robust mind and body, see my book, *Low Blood Sugar: A Doctor's Guide to Its Effective Control.* Your productive years will be prolonged by the effort and your life will be brighter.

Sludge and Disease

The anti-youth actions of sludging of your arteries and veins is so important that I believe it deserves separate discussion. I will discuss both sludging and disease states and how to overcome and prevent them for surging youth in subsequent chapters. Obviously, if you are to retain youth, the vital blood vessels carrying essential oxygen and energy to your body's organs, nerves and muscles must be kept freely open and in top functioning condition. There are also disease states which, if they are let go, will hasten aging. There are many other diseases that come and go and don't affect the aging process one way or the other. I'll discuss these with you and show you how to control them.

CHAPTER SUMMARY

1. Your body, your mind and your entire life are deeply affected by different kinds of cycles. To retard aging and retain youthful energy and sparkle, you need to control these cycles.
2. Your organic cycles involve bone, muscle, nerve, sex urge and many others. Careful attention to physical conditioning, body weight, diet, and alcohol ingestion will help you control your organic cycles and slow down the aging process.
3. Your body's blood sugar levels are vital. The correction of the factors that cause low blood sugar are easily managed and will assure an ample pool in your Fountain of Youth. Five simple rules of thumb aid you in this process.
4. The sex urge cycles of men and women aren't too different, and vary only slightly because of the menstrual

cycle in women. An understanding of what happens in sex cycles will enable you to live healthier, younger lives.

5. The environment you live in is likewise governed by cycles. Understanding the effects of weather, your job, your family, and the seasons helps you bring youth to the forefront.

6. The six anti-cycles and their effect on aging are under your control. If you bring them into phase, you will live a longer, happier, healthier life. Four of these anti-cycles have been discussed. The remaining two, sludge and disease, will be taken up in the next few sections.

6

How to De-sludge Your Arteries and Veins for a Youthfully Vital Body

If your body and your brain are to stay young, the tissues that make them up must be put in A-1 shape. The place to start this reconditioning process is with the vitally important arteries and veins that convey blood to and from these tissues. I will discuss with you in this section the way to keep your blood vessels in fine condition. I want to talk about how you can prevent your blood vessels from degenerating, hardening and becoming diseased; how you can prevent artery and vein occlusion (blockage) the most common killer and crippler of Americans today.

I want to talk about keeping your entire circulatory system in smooth, youthful and harmonious synchrony — your heart, your lungs, your vessels — how they can revitalize your organism and restore years of youthful life to your body and mind.

I'll also discuss with you what you can do when Nature makes a mistake; when one of the parts of your circulatory system is out of adjustment and isn't doing its full job for you.

I want to show you, in other words, how you can add years of youthfulness to the blood pumping and conveying system of your bodies: your heart, lungs and blood vessels.

HOW BLOOD VESSEL SLUDGE AGES YOU PREMATURELY

I don't think I need ask if you'd like to avoid having a coronary occlusion or a stroke. I'm sure you want no part of either one. Yet these two villians account for more deaths and disability among our citizens than any other disease! And why must we fall prey to these conditions? Why do we have to put up with them at all? The answer is all too simple, yet it defies explanation as to why heart disease and stroke remain the troublemakers they are today. Here's what happens:

1. A blood vessel carrying blood to heart muscle gets small "plaque" formations on its wall.
2. Large globs of fat and carbohydrate materials begin to cling to this plaque. Inflammatory reaction occurs around this area in blood vessel wall.
3. Over time, both inflammatory reaction and enlarging plaque with its "attractive" effect on material in blood going through it shut off more and more of the inside diameter of the blood vessel.
4. The heart muscle consequently doesn't get enough blood. The cause of coronary occlusion has been set up.

Of course, the rate at which this sludging develops varies a good deal. But even if the sludging rate in your arteries is slow, you will age faster than you should, and show it in your appearance and actions.

A PROGRAM TO REDUCE SLUDGE
IN YOUR BLOOD VESSELS

You can curb sludging in your arteries. And you can even cause sludge plaques that are already there to reduce in size — even disappear altogether! Remember, that it's the arteries that supply blood to your heart and brain that are of prime importance — they're small arteries to begin with, so small plaques in their walls are extremely dangerous. In the larger vessels, like the main artery that runs from your heart to your chest and abdomen — the aorta — small plaques are not of as great a consequence because the diameter inside such vessels is large. In these larger vessels, it is quite enough to just keep what plaques that are already there from getting any bigger.

Memorize these rules of thumb and put them in action curbing sludge in your arteries:

1. Reduce weight to ideal for your height and frame. (See tables at the end of this book.) Start reducing today!

2. Start an exercise routine today! Begin with any combination of toners I discussed in Chapter 3. Begin slowly. If you have a chronic illness, check your conditioning routine out with your doctor first.

3. If you have anyone in your immediate family tree who has had trouble with heart disease or stroke, let your doctor check your blood for too high cholesterol and fat levels. If these are of the kind not affected by diet (unusual, but not rare) start a routine prescribed by your doctor with a drug designed to lower the levels of these metabolic aliens to your blood stream. A special low cholesterol diet is printed in the appendix at the end of this book.

4. Avoid prolonged positions at home or at work that shut down the circulation to any arm or leg. Make it a habit to get up out of your chair at work at least six times a day and take a vigorous walk or jog or do some isometric exercises or anything to stir up your circulation.

5. Have your doctor treat any high blood pressure condition you may have. High blood pressure increases the rate of sludging in your vessels. The same is true of diabetes. And remember: physical exercise is known to help control diabetes!

HOW ED OVERCAME
SLUDGING HIS BLOOD VESSELS

One of the most unhappy men I can remember was Ed. Ed came to my office a shipwreck of a man. He was forty-six years old, looked fifty-six and felt sixty-six. Ed's circulation had become sludged to the point where, at the tender age of thirty-five years, he had his first coronary occlusion. Thirty-five is a young age indeed to think of having a coronary, but Ed did have one. When I received the records from his doctor in the town where he lived previously, the signs were there: sudden pain in the chest, feeling of crushing beneath his breast bone, feeling of suffocation and collapse at work one day out of a clear blue sky. Then followed three weeks in a hospital and six weeks away from work while his heart recovered.

Ed was fortunate in one respect. The size of his coronary was small and there were no complications in recovery. But

Ed was a "cripple." He was vastly overweight for his frame, suffered from angina of effort (pain in his chest on exertion) and the beginnings of sludging signs in his right leg. He couldn't walk more than half a city block without having intermittent claudication — a term meaning pain in the calf of his leg with exercise.

Ed began to recapture youth the day he started on a regime consisting of the following:

1. Reduction of his 234 pounds to ideal. In Ed's case, 165 pounds.
2. Starting a cholesterol-free diet. Fortunately, the kind of high cholesterol seen in most people is the kind that can be cured by avoiding cholesterol altogether. In the other cases, there are two or three good drugs that can reduce the fats in the blood stream to normal levels. One of these drugs is all that is usually necessary.
3. Following a *graduated* exercise routine. Ed was, of course, in no physical shape to start right off with vigorous exercising. He had too much disability from previous disease to be so foolhardy. Rather, I started him on slow daily toning routines only after his weight dropped about forty pounds — not yet an ideal level by any means, but enough to allow him to exert without angina (chest pain).

Today, Ed looks like a healthy, vigorous well-muscled man of about forty, even though he is actually fifty-one. He has completely lost his symptoms of leg pain when walking, and he can hike with the best of them. He hasn't had angina in four years. He has regained his youthful body by desludging his arteries.

HOW TO RECOVER FROM ANGINA

A patient of mine named Tom was more fortunate. His angina symptoms alerted him to impending trouble before he had a coronary occlusion. When I first saw Tom, he was forty-four years old. He had the typical build for a disastrous heart attack: overweight, flabby, short and squarely built and led a slothful life almost devoid of physical exercise and had a job in which was built the proposition that deadlines will be met even if it kills you! One day, Tom noted the sudden appearance of pressure beneath his breast bone. When he tried to move around, the pressure turned to a pain that seemed to shoot across the left side of his chest, into his shoulder and down the inside of his left arm. Tom was experiencing angina pectoris — chest pain from sludged heart muscle arteries.

What was happening in Tom's coronary arteries was a slow piling up of sludge — a gradual narrowing of the inside diameter of one of his coronary vessels. So much narrowing down had occurred that the area of heart muscle supplied by this artery wasn't getting enough vital oxygen. This lowered oxygen supply brought on his pain (angina). The following program helped Tom recover from his prematurely aging coronary vessels:

1. Reduction of weight. Tom was fifty-five pounds overweight for his height and frame.
2. A cholesterol-free diet (in addition to the usual reduction diet).
3. The use of a special drug that artificially dilates (makes bigger) coronary arteries. This got Tom rid of his angina completely and allowed him to increase his physical activity safely.
4. When Tom's weight had returned to near normal, I started him on *slow* isometric exercises. When he tolerated these well, I started some calisthenics — *slowly and gradually.* When he tolerated these well, I started him walking, then jogging every day. This gradual build-up of exercises took a period of a year. But today, Tom is off his medicine, He is trim, fit and physically in good shape. He hasn't had angina in a year and a half.

Tom's case illustrates the use of an extremely important tool in dealing with coronary arteries that are becoming sludged: *Besides preventing further artery occlusion, you can stop impending heart disease by forcing your body to increase the number of arteries that supply your heart with blood.* It is precisely this that Tom accomplished with his physical conditioning program!

REVERSING HIGH BLOOD PRESSURE

High blood pressure is caused by too much resistance to blood flow in arteries. The plaques and sludge I've already talked about can add to this problem, but the main cause of increased artery resistence is a tightening of the muscle coat that surrounds the artery. Eventually, the muscle layer around arteries becomes firm, rigid and unyielding. The result: hypertension or high blood pressure. There are other causes for abnormally high blood pressure — such other causes are rather unusual, but they need to be checked out. If there are no specific disease states causing high blood pressure, the condition is called essential hypertension — high blood pressure caused by too rigid a muscular coat around arteries.

HOW EDITH OVERCAME HYPERTENSION

And how do you cope with essential hypertension? Easy! Edith took care of hers as follows:

When I first saw Edith, a single career woman of forty years, she had begun to notice headaches of increasing severity, generalized chest pains, easy fatigability and dizzyness when getting out of a chair or bed.

In checking Edith over, I found her blood pressure to be 168/110. Definitely elevated for a woman of her age.

Some other facts came out in examining and talking with her. For instance, she was forty-eight pounds overweight, flabby and rather dumpy and she held a position characterized by a constant state of nervous tension because of the responsibilities associated with it. Further examination and tests over the following three days in the hospital revealed that she was free of heart disease and kidney disorder and her metabolism was normal. Fortunately for Edith, she had not yet developed the complications of sustained high blood pressure. She looked about fifteen years older than her forty years, however, and would have undoubtedly succumbed to complications of her diseased arteries at an early date had she not taken her trouble in hand.

I had a long chat with Edith after I was satisfied she was free of complications. I told her that first and foremost, she must get her weight down and keep it there if she was to obtain a cure. She told me of repeated past attempts to control her weight without avail. I next discussed with her the role of her mind in her high blood pressure. How her constant nervous state had to be overcome and how she could use the power of mind to help her do this. She was not impressed.

"Are you telling me I can will away my troubles, Doctor?" she asked.

"Not exactly," I replied, "but you can use concentration and suggestion to learn to relax."

Edith did learn. She also discovered the benefits of physical conditioning in helping both her elevated blood pressure and her relaxing.

For a while, Edith took a single drug to control her blood pressure while she got at the crux of her problem. Within four months, she had lost twenty-five pounds, had begun to tone up soft flabby muscles and could sleep without a sedative or tranquilizer, two of her mainstays before this time. After another six months, Edith lost another twenty-three pounds, was able to stop the blood pressure medicine altogether and looked and felt twenty years younger than a year before! Today, Edith remains in the pink of health and enjoys the youth she'd almost let slip by. She has also very probably averted a stroke in the process!

HOW JOYCE OVERCAME HER STROKE

The term stroke means either a rupture or a narrowing down of the blood vessels in the brain. Stroke is the counterpart of a coronary in the heart. Both can be avoided, because what I've already said about blood vessels in the heart apply as well to your brain. But what if you've already had a stroke — is it possible to regain a reasonably normal mind and body again? Most certainly!

Joyce had given up the ship entirely following a stroke. In Joyce's case, one of the main arteries in the right side of her brain underwent an occlusion and suddenly Joyce found herself paralyzed on the left side, unable to control her bladder or bowel and partially blind in her right eye. She was able to speak fairly well — the speech center in the brain is usually located on the left side of the brain in right handed people. If her stroke had been in an artery on the left side of her brain, she would probably have lost the ability to talk as well.

Joyce was one of the fortunate ones. The medicine she took to help prevent further extension of the blood clot, probably stuck to a large plaque inside the artery wall, worked well and eventually the clot absorbed. Over a period of three months, Joyce regained the ability to use her left arm and leg, regained control of her bladder and bowels and could see fairly well from her partially blinded eye.

When she was feeling fairly well, I told her she could expect another stroke again, when, no one could say, but it would come — unless she began immediate steps to prevent it.

Of course, she was willing to do anything to prevent another such episode. Joyce was in her mid-fifties and not a whole lot overweight — no more than twenty pounds or so. This was easily gotten rid of. Her blood pressure was moderately elevated, about 170/100 most of the time. A single drug sufficed to bring this down to normal. Her cholesterol levels were unusually high, however, and I discovered that the main reason for this was that she had a definitely underactive thyroid gland, the gland that directs the rate cells in your body to burn up energy. This was corrected by adding thyroid extract to her daily routine. Soon, her cholesterol returned to normal levels. At this time, Joyce started graduated physical conditioning. She was able to come along rapidly with these and now wouldn't start or end the day without doing fifteen to twenty-five minutes of various toning exercises. Five years later, Joyce hasn't had any further strokes. She has added at least ten years to her life!

HOW NATURE'S MISTAKES MAY BE REPAIRED

Every now and again, Nature makes an error in turning out hearts and blood vessels. Sometimes, the error is in the formation of the heart walls as it was in Roy's case when I first saw him with his parents in the office one day. It seems Roy was on the high school wrestling team and noted increasing shortness of breath. Work-up indicated Roy had a small hole between the two upper chambers of his heart. During development of the fetus, a hole normally appears in this area, but closes before birth. Roy's hadn't.

Three months following surgical repair of this hole, Roy was back wrestling on the team.

A young lady of twenty-one I know was also born with a "mistake." This time, the mistake was in the large artery leaving the left ventricle (lower chamber) of the heart — the aorta. It had a "pinch" in it just beyond its emergence from the heart as it arches downward into the chest. The pinch was causing elevated blood pressure in Dawn's arms; lowered blood pressure in her legs (below the "pinch") and strain on her heart muscle. Her youthful days were numbered!

One month after repair of the "pinch" (it was excised and the large vessel sewn together) Dawn could look forward to fifty more years of normal healthy life again.

HOW RHEUMATIC FEVER EFFECTS
WERE OVERCOME

This once dreaded heart crippler is also coming under the gun of the surgeon. Acute rheumatic fever is caused by an allergic reaction to a certain strain of streptococcus bacteria — the kind that causes "strep" throat and some other infections. Because the system develops an allergic response to the peculiar protein of this germ, certain of the body's cells react violently to it. Among these cells are those lining the heart chambers, especially the heart valves between the four chambers. When this happens, the valves can be irreparably damaged — the so-called rheumatic heart — causing leakage of the heart. Incomplete closing and opening of the valve is involved.

The last youngster of fifteen years I saw with a severely damaged mitral valve (the one between the left auricle and ventricle in the heart) was so incapacitated from his valve disease that he was confined to a wheel chair. His life expectancy was about ten more years if he were lucky. And if you could call such a thing as Tommy had a life!

Tommy is alive, kicking and looking forward to three score and ten healthy years now as a result of an operation that completely replaced the damaged mitral valve. He can never become a professional mountain climber or a distance track runner, but can do just about everything else he wants to, thanks to the skills of surgery.

CHAPTER SUMMARY

1. Sludged arteries and veins cause rapid aging. De-sludging can restore years of vigorous useful life to your organism. Start today to prevent sludging from occurring. If it has already started, you can take the necessary steps to halt the process.
2. Your entire blood vessel system, including your heart, will stay younger longer with proper attention to the problem of sludge.
3. High blood pressure and strokes are no barrier to de-sludging activities on your part. Started today, the de-sludging process may very well prevent you from having either one of these cripplers.
4. Very few heart conditions today, even if they've progressed to advanced stages, cannot be improved or cured with the skilled surgeon's scalpel. Following this correction, you can start your blood vessels on their way to younger, vital lives.

7

How to Charge Vital,
Youth-Building Energy
into Your Organs
and Nerves

In this chapter, I want to show you the dynamics of your body's energy turnover and how to avoid some of the things that can upset it. I want to acquaint you with your body electricity and how to keep it from getting grounded out. Yes, I said your body electricity! Of course your body doesn't have quite the jolt that the electric light plugs in your house have, but your body does, nevertheless, depend on small electric currents to do its job. I want you to understand how this works as far as your nerves are concerned so that you'll be able to keep your nervous system young and in top working order.

I want to talk about the disorders of this body electricity and how you can reverse the rigors of such disorders and regain a youthful nervous system once again.

Your brain consists of roughly thirteen billion tiny cells that make up, among other things, your mind. When the electric power plants in these cells go haywire, you can have all kinds of aging mind trouble. I want to show how to prevent this from happening, and how to deal with it if it should happen.

HOW YOUTHFULNESS DEPENDS ON
ENERGY CONTROL

Your whole organism depends upon a constant and well-regulated supply of energy to keep it functioning smoothly. You can liken this situation to a power generating plant — as long as the dynamos in the plant are fed a continuing supply of energy, and as long as the dynamos' parts are kept in top running condition, the power outflow from the plant hums along nicely and at a constant rate. But let anything interrupt this flow of energy to the dynamos — the power output goes down accordingly. Your body is the same. What is it in the human organism that's so vital to its cells (dynamos)? It's *sugar and oxygen*. Both these ingredients are absolutely necessary for body cells to continue their uninterrupted function.

Nerve cells are particularly vulnerable to a drop of supply in either of these two ingredients. Haven't you noticed that one of the first things that happens when you allow your blood sugar to drop (go too long between meals, for instance) is that you get jittery, jumpy and nervous? When the oxygen supply is diminished or cut off, what's the first thing that happens? You get drowsy and finally lapse into unconsciousness. Nerve cells must have a constant ready supply of both sugar and oxygen for their function.

HOW A DISASTER OF LOW BODY
ELECTRICITY WAS AVERTED

An example of letting energy reserves dwindle to dangerous levels was seen in a patient I'll call Kate. Kate was really asking for trouble and I'm afraid she got it. Fortunately, she came back, and retrieved about fifteen years of youth in the process. Kate came to me complaining of complete lack of pep and energy. She was a "blimp" type, with 180 pounds packed on a five foot five inch frame. She had resolved herself to a life of complete sluggishness and lack of contact with the outside world, so great was her withdrawal of energy. Her complexion was sallow, she had high blood pressure, she had swollen ankles and soreness in almost every joint and muscle in her body.

She did eat, though. And denied any overeating! I asked her how she managed to pack sixty excess pounds on her frame if she didn't eat any more than she claimed. "Why, all my people are large, doctor," she said, as though she were doomed to this state because of her grandparents' and uncles' and aunts' follies.

I put Kate in the hospital and in checking her response to a measured amount of glucose (sugar) I found she had hypo-glycemia — low blood sugar. She was starving her nerve cells of vital functioning while becoming a pig in appearance in the process! It was really no use arguing a daily diet program with Kate. She'd been through the "diet mill." Instead, I imposed a 600 calorie a day diet on her while she was in the hospital. In less than a week, Kate lost fifteen pounds. (I also kept her quite active through the good efforts of the physiotherapy department who agreed to work Kate out in their department twice a day.)

When Kate saw that she could indeed lose weight through effective dieting, I was able to continue her routine at home.

She was able to do a better job when I explained to her that hypoglycemia was, in a patient with her build and background, only one step this side of having diabetes — the condition where blood sugar builds up to extremely high levels, there being no insulin in her body system to burn it up. This spurred Kate into eating purposefully for weight reduction. She began to reduce her intake of calories, to eat six small meals a day instead of gorging at three large ones, to have a high protein, moderate fat, low carbohydrate intake, begin to maintain a twice daily exercise routine built on isometrics and jogging, and to learn mind control to help with diet exercising and getting out of the mental stupor she'd fallen into.

Within seven months, Kate's blood sugar returned to normal and I hardly knew her as the same slovenly fat person she'd once been. She regained a bright, attentive alert look. She became interested in what was going on. And most of all Kate rejoined the ranks of wife and mother to her family, much to the delight of Kate's husband and children.

ENERGY CONTROL MEANS POSITIVE METABOLISM

What is positive metabolism? Consider the events that follow:

1. Sugar is absorbed into your system. Delivered via blood stream to cell for metabolism.
2. Insulin acts on sugar enabling it to be burned to carbon dioxide (waste product of all metabolism) and water.
3. Oxygen released from (2) above, enters cell machinery as "fuel." Carbon dioxide is expelled, enters blood stream and carried to lungs where it is exhaled.

When this sequence is running along smoothly, efficiently and constantly, you have positive metabolism. Anything that disrupts this flow causes negative metabolism.

How Burt Regained His Youth-fulness Reversing Negative Metabolism

A dramatic experience by a patient named Burt shows how youth can be deftly snatched back from oblivion by simply reversing negative metabolism. Burt came to me originally with all the signs and symptoms of hyperlipemia — just a long word meaning too much fat in the blood stream. He literally had fat dissolved in his blood to the point that if the lab drew a specimen of his blood and allowed it to stand for a minute in a small test tube, the serum portion (the part left over when the red blood cells settle to the bottom) was pure cream in appearance!

Burt was well on his way to seventy-five years at the tender age of thirty. Already he was having angina pectoris (chest pains resulting from partially occluded or blocked coronary arteries), fatty deposits around his eyes (usually seen only in senility), fatty tumors scattered in large clumps around his body, lethargy, listlessness, and impending diabetes. His cells were starved for energy even though it was flowing in pure form through his blood stream!

Burt had the kind of lipemia considered caused by an hereditary defect. That is, his genes were somehow abnormal. A certain drug can reverse this process in most people. It did in Burt's case. Thyroid extract speeded up his slow metabolism when it was found to be quite low. The thyroid also helped lower his blood fat level. Diet and exercise got Burt back on the metabolic track and finally conquered his angina pectoris as well.

Today, Burt has normal blood fats, has perfectly functioning metabolism, and has averted serious heart disease, blood vessel disease with possible occlusion of a brain or major limb (arm or leg) artery. And most importantly, Burt has turned back his biological clock which was running at an incredible speed to age him prematurely!

HOW NEGATIVE ENTROPY
AFFECTS YOUTHFULNESS

Physicists have shown that a condition called *entropy* exists in any closed system (an independently operating unit). The exact definition of entropy isn't so important as much as its general meaning: the energy that's *unavailable* to the system's operation. As far as your body cells are concerned, entropy means the energy that's tied up in maintaining the status quo — the power potential or integrity of the cell as opposed to energy available to do the *work* of the cell.

Life depends on an abundance of *negative entropy.* That is, a condition in the trillions of body cells where most of the energy is available to do work. If it were not for this condition, the very complex molecules making up the cells' insides would quickly deteriorate into their basic atoms — carbon, oxygen, nitrogen and hydrogen — and life as we know it would cease to exist.

Keeping cells in this state of negative entropy is a tremendously complex task for your metabolism. Energy control helps with this giant accomplishment for youthful health.

Aging, in fact, is just such a loss of negative entropy with either a gradual or sudden slip to positive entropy — a condition where most of the available energy must be used just to keep the cell from deteriorating. It follows that the more a cell goes toward positive entropy, the more its building blocks of life deteriorate into its basic atoms — *the more, in other words, the cell ages.* Carried on a little further, positive entropy ends in the death of cells, and the body's inability to repair or replace them.

MAN THROWS CHAINS OF POSITIVE ENTROPY

When I first saw Chad, he was well on his way out of the picture from alcoholism. He was the picture of the aging senile man at his true age of forty-nine.

He had been a habitual alcoholic for about twelve years, and the health toll had been heavy upon him. Chad's liver, for example, was enlarged that it occupied fully half of his abdominal cavity (it normally occupies about a fourth of it).

He had muscle wasting in his arms and legs, and was about thirty-five pounds underweight.

Chad was beginning to have difficulty coordinating his muscles to do what he wanted them to in just getting around. He was not burning his sugar properly, and this was bad news. Chad was in positive entropy.

Interestingly enough, it wasn't until Chad's energy turnover was corrected that he began to show signs of recovering — of getting back to negative entropy. In the hospital, I began Chad's treatment with a substance called fructose given intravenously and in concentrated amounts. I used fructose (a sugar-like substance that doesn't depend on insulin for its metabolism) because I knew giving glucose (plain sugar) would further aggravate his already low sugar levels. The reason for this is as follows:

1. Low levels of circulating sugar plus inability of liver to respond adequately to stimulation to release what stores it may have.
2. Sugar given. Stimulates pancreas which is already exhausted. Pancreas responds with insufficient insulin (needed to burn sugar).
3. Only fraction of sugar burned. Rest metabolized incompletely or not at all causing further disruption and negative metabolism.
4. Energy turnover worse than before because still insufficient glucose and improperly metabolized substances adding to waste disposal problem.

Once Chad had his reserves of quick energy built up so his cells had enough to do their normal jobs, his liver could begin to store glucose for future use. When his liver began to function again, I placed him on a high protein, moderate carbohydrate and low fats diet that returned his positive entropy to the negative side — gave his cells enough to work with for the repair of their damage *plus their normal work.*

Once this was accomplished, Chad was ready for muscle toning, an activity for which he wasn't mentally ready, but for which he was conditioned by practicing mind control with autosuggestion and concentration.

In time, Chad began his long trip back to normal. Within fourteen months, Chad regained his weight and ten pounds of additional solid muscle. He was encouraged to remain on the wagon through the good graces of Alcoholics Anonymous. He began literally to lose years from his body and mind to the extent that he now looks about five years younger than he did at the start. Proof positive that given half the chance, your body and mind can, indeed, accomplish the impossible!

YOUR YOUTH PHASE AND
HOW TO KEEP IT WORKING

Your body electricity generated by those trillions of individual dynamos, the cells, must be kept in phase if you are to remain young. How is this done? The following should not only be committed to memory, but should *be practiced every day*:

1. Keep your body and mind in harmony. If you've been putting something off in restoring a part of parts of your body to health, don't put it aside any longer — deliver it to your doctor and have it fixed — NOW.
2. Get off your mind anything that's "stuck" there. Anything that's eating you, bugging you, making you miserable — get to the source of the problem and end it here and now.
3. Start getting your body weight in conformity with your height and frame now.
4. Start your conditioning routines, first thing in the morning and last thing at night, today.
4. Put the reservoirs of your mind at your disposal instead of letting them stagnate. Mobilize your powers of concentration, autosuggestion and will and train them to work for you starting today.
6. Adjust your living cycles so that you feel comfortable and relaxed while working with them. If one or more of your cycles are off, readjust to work in harmony with the rest of your organism today.

HOW MENTAL ILLNESS AND RESULTANT AGING
IS A MATTER OF CELL ELECTRICITY

If there were ever a reason for alarm in our country's health today, in addition to the usually listed "top ten" diseases, I'm convinced that it lies in the realm of mental illness. One hears a good deal about how large mental institutions have reduced their patient load or have "eliminated the back ward" and so on. This makes things look good on the surface, but hardly conceals the fact that the only reason such reductions and eliminations have been possible is because of the advent of the potent new tranquilizers. These drugs have quieted down patients that a decade or so ago would have been "climbing the walls" in padded cells or in straight jackets. Currently, the number of people in dire need of help with mental health problems is increasing rapidly. Today more of them are dealt with on an outpatient basis whereas formerly, they would had to have been placed in institutions.

What happens when a person "goes off the deep end" mentally? The whole answer isn't known, unfortunately. But it's being worked on in research areas throughout the country. Suffice to say, something happens to cause the mind to become completely disrupted from its usual framework. Whether cause or effect, there are physical and chemical changes that occur when this happens.

One of these changes is in the electrical activity, not of individual cells, but in large clones — clusters or groups — of cells. The electroencephalogram, a machine used to record the electrical activity of cells in the brain, are incapable of picking such disturbances up. Hence, the EEG patterns of the mentally disturbed are not altered unless the cells happen to have other disease as well.

HOW A MENTAL PATIENT REGAINED
HER YOUTHFULNESS

I first met Lila as a patient in a mental institution. Lila was thirty-eight when she was admitted to the mental hospital. She had a very unhappy traumatic childhood and her marriage had ended in divorce. Without going into the sordid details of Lila's early life, she began to have hallucinations and delusions of persecution shortly after the divorce. This means she saw things that weren't there and had bizarre ideas pop up in her head with absolutely no basis in fact and for no justifiable reason.

When she was first admitted for intensive care, she was completely unable to give a rational coherent history. She looked like a tramp. She was filthy dirty, disheveled, and smelled like a sewer. She was literally living in a world of her own, having no contact with reality except to regard everything and everybody as her enemy.

Shortly after her admission to the hospital, she calmed down through the benefit of drugs that caused her to stop hallucinating. Gradually, she began to take some interest in herself, cleaned up, dressed appropriately and neatly and came to regard other people as not against her.

When Lila was ready to try going out into the real world once again, she came into my office with a minor complaint. While talking to her, I suggested that she might utilize the principles of youth-building to regain some of her lost years — she still looked fifteen years older than her actual age. She was eager to try.

As she progressed with her weight problem, her exercises, her cycle and mind rejuvenation and her energy turnover phases, she told me that she felt she might be able to do with less of the powerful tranquilizers she had been maintained on since coming out of the hospital. A talk with her psychiatrist was met with much skepticism, however. He was concerned she might regress and start the whole process all over again, losing all she'd gained. So we agreed not to alter the medicine. The patient had other ideas, however. Lila, on her own, began to reduce the medicine. Gradually at first, with several weeks between reductions. With each reduction, she redoubled her efforts with her youth program.

Finally, she weaned herself off medicines entirely. She remained well, happy and found a new life with her youth program and with a new marriage. Lila isn't perfect — few of us are. But for a year and a half now, she's remained off medicines and free of mental crippling. I think this says something for her youth program: that when mentally ill persons reach a certain stage in their progress through psychiatric and drug help, then picking up with the use of one's *own resources* may greatly aid in preventing further breakdown. Hopefully, someday soon we may find a good practical answer to the dilemma of mentally ill people. Meanwhile, a sound youth-building program may help many of them.

HOW A VICTIM OF EPILEPSY PROFITED FROM A YOUTH BUILDING PROGRAM

I'd like to mention briefly that epilepsy — often termed "fits" or seizures — need not be a hindrance to youth building. Like so many other disease processes, I've noticed that people with epilepsy do better and have less trouble when they pursue a good youth-building program.

Tracy, a young woman I know very well, is a good example. When I first met her, she had become a "household invalid" — a term I've coined for epileptics who've become convinced that they must live a life of seclusion at home because of the "cross they bear."

When Tracy embarked on her program of weight control, muscle toning and mind control, she changed into a completely different person just as sweet and lovely as any young girl you'd want to know. She started the program only after the greatest of persuasion. She was completely doubtful of positive results. It was only when she saw what a difference a few exercises made in her drab daily life that she agreed to go ahead with more youth-building. Of course, Tracy still takes medicine to prevent seizures. She has been able to reduce these medicines twice since starting her program without the occurrence of a single seizure. She will probably always have to use some medicine. But she will have gained twenty years of happiness by letting herself grow young rather than prematurely old, without ever having really known what spiritual uplifting can be accomplished by one's self!

CHAPTER SUMMARY

1. Proper energy turnover is essential to youth. Your energy turnover can be altered to furnish your cells with vital youth-giving fuel.
2. Proper restoration of energy turnover can prevent disease — even reverse that which may already be started.

3. The tiny building blocks inside the trillions of your cells must have energy to spare for youthfulness in addition to what it takes just to keep the cell in working order. To reach this state of ideal "negative entropy" your organism must be put in phase and harmony with all its parts.

4. Your youth-building program, consisting of weight control, exercise routines, mind mastery, cycle control and adequate energy input, helps insure your organism of long-lasting, vigorous youthfulness.

8

How to Build a Youthful Digestive and Elimination System in Your Body

Since that area between tongue and anus has to do both with digestion and elimination, and since proper digestion of food helps your cells stay young, I want to discuss this system with you and show you how to keep it in youthful working order.

The stomach and intestines are your body's "sounding board" of excess nervous energy. An understanding of this state of affairs and how to reverse it will help you restore your youthfulness.

Your digestive glands have to last all your life. You need to know how to keep them functioning youthfully. These glands, too, are subject to a variety of insults. You can avoid the penalties of these insults if you know what to expect. We'll talk about how this is done in this chapter.

The urinary system is another important waste eliminator system in your body. It is' subject to a variety of disorders, most of which you can navigate around. You will be shown how to accomplish this.

The skin is, believe it or not, one of your body's most important organs of elimination as well as being the prime organ of temperature regulation for you. Its care for youth-building, therefore, is vital. I'll discuss this important organ in this section also.

HOW AN AGING GASTROINTESTINAL SYSTEM TURNED ON FOR YOUTHFULNESS AGAIN

Emma's GI system was sluggish. As a consequence, Emma was aging far before her time. (The term "GI" stands for gastrointestinal — commonly, the stomach and bowel). Emma complained of stuffiness, gas and bloating. She belched all the time and had vague pains shooting all over her abdomen, especially after meals. She was fat, dumpy and had myriad complaints in addition to those in her GI system. All this finally progressed to the point of bowel difficulties, with the appearance of flatuousness (passing of excess rectal gas), difficult greasy and unpredictable bowel movements, and signs of poor absorption or assimilation into her system of foods she ate.

Emma was miserable and had been on a dozen or more "special" diets and had taken twice this many "stomach and bowel medicines" in order to try and straighten out her misbehaving intestinal works. All these were to no avail, and Emma had become convinced that she needed "surgery or something" to make her well.

"The only surgery that might help you at this time," I said to her one day, "is a radical removal of the fat hanging down from your abdominal wall." Emma wasn't pleased with this comment. "Well," she replied, "if that's what it takes, that's what I'll have done!" And she stormed out of the office. She returned, however, a little later in the week, mostly to complain about her nagging aches and pains again. Finally, I said to her, "Do you *really* want to feel better again? Would you like to restore your GI system to its former efficient self again and add about fifteen years to your life and look much younger in the process?" Emma was speechless for a minute, then a smile crossed her face. "Who wouldn't?" she asked, laughing aloud. Here's the schedule Emma followed:

1. I put Emma on a low residue diet. This is a dietary routine that leaves as little possible for the intestine to have to evacuate as waste. A typical low residue diet is included in the appendix at the end of the book.
2. I took Emma *off all her drugs.* I did put her on a suppository insertion program that stimulates the muscle coat of the lower bowel. I had her use this every night.
3. I started Emma on vigorous calisthenics program also over her protestations, including sit-ups. She was otherwise healthy and had no past history of trouble, so she could stand the pressure of exercise.

For the next four weeks, I listened to Emma complain bitterly about the routine. She grumbled and complained loudly. She begged. She wept. But I told her if she wanted help from me, she must cooperate absolutely and without compromise. The next four weeks saw fewer complaints and more improvement. Emma had reached the first plateau: she found out for herself that she "had it in her" to remedy her sluggish GI tract. The gassiness and bloating disappeared rather rapidly, since the diet didn't allow any food that could form gas if it were properly chewed during meal time.

Emma found that the main reason for her belching was something she was doing unconsciously in addition to her atrocious dietary habits: She was an air-swallower. She enjoyed gorging herself so much and was so upset from long neglect of body that she was unconsciously swallowing air with all her stuffing of food! The air she swallowed was trapped in her stomach and had nowhere to go but up. And up it came in the form of recurrent belching.

When she became used to her muscle toning routine, I eliminated the suppository. She found that her "training" produced results in the form of regular bowel movements every other night without further use of laxatives.

Finally, when she had completely straightened her GI system out, Emma began to lose weight, learn control of her mind and return from the land of premature old age. Today, Emma looks and feels as though she had lost age as well as weight. She hasn't had GI complaints in over two years.

NERVE CONTROL ESSENTIAL TO YOUTHFUL GI SYSTEM

Of all the ills that age your GI system, your nerves are number one on the list. It's long been recognized that a pair of large nerves, called the vagus nerves, that lead from your brain to your stomach and bowel are the channels over which much excess nervous energy is diverted. This is your mind's safety valve. When the pressure builds up for whatever reason, your mind has to let off the steam, so to speak. It does this in a number of ways, but that done through the vagus nerves is a very common one.

When this happens, all hell may break loose as far as your GI system is concerned. There is virtually no symptom that nerves, being used in this way, cannot produce. I'm not saying that *all* GI symptoms are thus produced, but the majority of them are. The chief cause of stomach ulcers, for instance, is nervous imbalance of this sort. Ben found this out and profited from his knowledge.

Ben first appeared in the emergency room of a hospital hemorrhaging profusely from ulcers. About 90 percent of 'stomach ulcers' are actually located in the first twelve inches of the small intestine just beyond the stomach. The other 10 percent are in the stomach proper. When an ulcer bleeds from its more usual location, that is in the intestine, beyond the stomach, the bleeding usually appears as tarry, black-looking stools in addition to the usual pain and heartburn that accompanies most ulcers. That is just what Ben was experiencing.

He was a man in his twenties, held a good job and had a family. In talking to Ben later, I found that he was one of those kind of people who take everything and everybody far too seriously; who works under a terrific burden of their own *assumed* responsibility even though they may have very little *real* responsibility; who constantly stew and fret about family problems, friends, the world situation in general and who really never learned proper ways of getting rid of these terrific heads of built-up steam in any other way but to "keep them inside."

When Ben was well on his way to recovery from the bleeding episode, which incidentally stopped of its own accord, we began to talk about how to get over this "carrying the cross" attitude. I told Ben truthfully that if he didn't learn how to do this, he would likely end up having surgery with removal of part or all his stomach and the many troubles that often follow such surgery. He agreed that something had to be done.

Ben began his recovery by learning an alternate way for his organism to vent the steam heads that developed in his mind: that of vigorous exercising at least twice a day and more often when he felt particularly "tight" and tense. In addition to regular physical workouts, Ben got hold of a punching bag and joined a hand ball unit at his neighborhood YMCA. Now, when Ben feels like "getting something off his chest" he either works up a real sweat at the punching bag or plays a set or two of handball until he gets rid of all his pent-up emotional strain. In addition, Ben has learned that there are some things that stomach ulcers simply will not tolerate via the diet. A list of these items is in the appendix at the end of the book. He takes neither medicines nor special pains with his diet today, and has not had further trouble with ulcers.

THE NERVOUS STOMACH ELIMINATED

A young woman named Jan probably saved herself an early grave by heading off ulcerative colitis, a complication of a nervous gut that may enter the picture if allowed to progress unchecked. Jan began to have diarrhea and cramps with a little bleeding and mucous in her bowel movements. Taking medicines and diet slowed down the process, but the symptoms persisted. Jan was an intelligent career woman who had, for reasons not important to our discussion, become a very dependent person — someone who needed constant support in everything she did. The excess nervous energy from such dependence was shunted over the nerves to her GI tract with the results mentioned above.

The first thing I taught Jan was to substitute a potent emotional tool for her dependence. Jan happened to be interested in the field of music, but hadn't followed through with it. She learned to play the organ. In time, this substitution therapy worked as a good intestinal soother — it was a *creative* activity, helped her avert immeasurable grief and restored youth to her GI system.

HOW TO AVOID GALLBLADDER DISEASE

No discussion of an aging GI system would be complete without mention of the gall bladder, a small muscular sac beneath the liver that stores bile for digestion of certain foods. Remember the following points about your gall bladder to keep it from aging you prematurely:

1. Keep your weight at *ideal* levels. For every one person I've seen with gall stones who was of lean build, I've seen a hundred who have been grossly overweight.

2. Keep your dietary fats on the low side. Trim fat off meat before eating it; avoid the use of butter, cream, gravies and oils; avoid rich pastries and confections and keep your alcohol intake at sensible levels.
3. Keep physically active!

PROGRAM FOR ITCHING RUMP SYNDROME

Sometimes the GI system will remain in good shape except for the sudden onset, for no apparent reason, of severe unremitting itching around the rectum. Many things are blamed for this distressing situation. But generally none of the commonly incriminated factors are to blame. It's usually caused from the exactly same thing that causes diarrhea, cramps and bloating — nerves. The following program will usually cause this aggravating symptom to stop:

1. Keep everything off the itching skin for a short time. This means soap, water, medicines, etc. Use only mineral oil on cotton to clean the area following bowel movements. Nothing else.
2. Take twelve to sixteen Brewer's yeast tablets daily with meals. These can be purchased at the drug store without a prescription and are quite inexpensive.
3. Stop all medicines and drugs that aren't absolutely necessary.
4. Go on the same low residue diet that's listed on the appendix of the book until the problem is cleared up.
5. Use mind control to help. (At night, for example, concentrate on the itching area to become numb.) Eliminate any source of personal trouble such as hostility to spouse or boss, sexual frustrations and other emotionally upsetting situations.

MAINTAINING A YOUTHFUL URINARY SYSTEM

Your kidneys and their collecting systems, the bladder and urethra (the tube that discharges urine from the bladder) form a vitally important elimination function. The lower part of the human urinary system is closely bound up with the reproductive system. Sometimes, trouble in one will reflect itself by symptoms in the other and vice versa.

Kidneys

These organs are the great filters of your blood system. They're important enough that Nature has provided each person with two of them, though under usual circumstances a part of just one is enough to sustain health. There is no such thing as "straining" a kidney — they're quite up to most anything in the way of increased load you can push at them. It's the opposite, the lack of a load, that may often prove injurious to kidneys. To keep your kidneys youthful and prevent them from aging prematurely, the following points are important:

1. *Always* drink plenty of fluids. You need more when the weather's hot and after you exercise. It's quite difficult to drink too much fluid; it's easy not to drink enough.
2. If you work at a job that works up a sweat, drink even more fluid. The majority of urinary tract infections start as a result of making your kidneys concentrate your urine in a small volume of fluid, thereby allowing organisms normally present in urine to overgrow and start infection.
3. Follow a vigorous physical activity program. The more blood circulated through the kidneys, the better they remove waste products from your body. Keep your weight down! Flab increases the load on kidneys and causes changes to take place in them that may herald high blood pressure.
4. Have everything that's wrong with your *lower* urinary system corrected immediately and without delay. In women, for example, a bladder that's allowed to flop back in the pelvis because of poor muscular support as a result of having children predisposes to infection and stasis of urine. Eventually, this damages kidneys. In men, for example, an enlarging prostate gland obstructs the flow of urine from the bladder and causes the same trouble. You can't afford to prematurely age kidneys by

neglecting their proper drainage. Have such trouble corrected immediately!

WHEN KIDNEY TROUBLE STRIKES

Iris allowed her trouble to go unchecked. She ended up with chronic kidney damage as a result. She began to notice recurrent episodes of burning during urination, urgency to get to the bathroom quickly or dribble urine if she didn't, a feeling of never quite emptying her bladder even though she "squeezed all the urine out she felt was there."

Iris had four children and was not one to engage in physical conditioning. Her muscles were all flabby as a result, including those whose function it is to firm up and support the pelvic organs and rectum.

She began to have mild lower urinary infections which were treated successfully with antibiotics. Eventually, however, in spite of repeated warnings to have the necessary repair work done, Iris' infections began to involve her kidneys. She ended up with a chronic kidney condition that damaged their ability to filter properly.

Iris finally got the repair work done to her lower pelvis and has had no further trouble with her bladder control or with urine infections. Her kidneys continue to allow a small amount of the protein in her blood stream to leak out in her urine. (Normally, no protein should come into the urine.) They're unable to concentrate her urine as they once were so that she has to take in an added amount of fluid every day. She must eat more protein to compensate for the loss through her kidneys. Now, it's even more important than ever that Iris follow a youth-building program. She can live a normal, healthy life if she continues to maintain adequate and ideal weight and if she continues to get reasonable exercise and physical activity. Thus far, that's just what she's doing. And I believe Iris will do well in spite of the damage her kidneys have sustained.

A YOUTHFUL PROSTATE

In men, prostate trouble can begin to appear any time after forty-five or so. It usually comes on later, but not necessarily. The following list of factors aggravate the prostate gland —

cause it to enlarge. And because of its peculiar position — the gland virtually surrounds the urethra — any enlargement will tend to close off this tube leading from the bladder to the outside:

1. Venereal diseases. The bacteria that causes venereal disease irritates and inflames the prostate. Given enough irritation, the prostate will enlarge.
2. Too much or too little sexual activity will irritate the prostate and cause it to enlarge. A good argument in favor of a "middle of the road" viewpoint in sexual contacts.
3. Too little exercise, especially with later years, causes natural secretions to collect in the prostate gland instead of being emptied out as they are in the usual course of events. This causes enlargement.
4. Repeated lower urinary (bladder) infections.

Frank, a patient with such trouble, noted increasing difficulty starting his urine. He also noticed that he began to get up to urinate a lot at night even though he tried to cut his fluids down in the latter part of day. He noted some dribbling of urine — some loss of urine between times in the bathroom. His prostate was enlarging.

Frank's urologist recommended a TUR. A TUR is a surgical procedure in which the enlarged prostate tissue is removed with an instrument from within the urethra. When this was done, Frank no longer had any of his symptoms. He was able to control his urine, he had no more bladder infections and there was no diminuation of his sexual activities. He saved himself much potential grief later when a more radical procedure would undoubtedly have to have been done. Frank regained his youthful urinary system by not ignoring or postponing action on signs of trouble.

CHAPTER SUMMARY

1. You can have a youthful digestive and elimination system by utilizing the principles of control: physical conditioning and mind control.

2. Most digestive disease is caused from poor control of excess nervous energy. Your mind is the key to eliminating this trouble.
3. Your urinary system is vitally important to body waste elimination. If you follow a program of youth-building for your urinary system, you may avoid serious consequences in the future.

9

Secrets of an Effective Breathing Method to Promote Youthfulness

The air you breathe and how you breathe it may mean the difference between extended youth or premature aging. I will talk about this important activity in this section.

I want to discuss with you the question of emphysema and asthma. I want you to learn how to prevent both these cripplers that can age you before your time, and to tell you what to do when they appear for you.

The subject of air pollution is with us today. I want to discuss with you how to keep your lungs unpolluted and how to depollute them if they've already become contaminated.

Inasmuch as your heart is so much bound up with your breathing system, you should know how to keep this blood pump in youthful condition and vital good health at all times.

Your blood's prime function is to carry the essential oxygen you breathe in. I will talk about how to keep it from becoming stale and old even after your 70th birthday.

YOUR OXYGEN REJUVENATION SYSTEM

Every hour without realizing it, you inhale about 300-400 gallons of air. This air contains oxygen, nitrogen and carbon dioxide in addition to other ingredients. Oxygen is the vital constituent as far as your life is concerned.

When oxygen gets into the lungs, it passes through an unbelievably thin membrane separating your lung air sacs from your blood stream. Once in the bloodstream, oxygen is loosely "bound" to hemoglobin, the red pigment of your blood, where it is carried along with other vital nutrients to your body cells. At the cell, oxygen is "released" from this hemoglobin bond where it diffuses into the cell. When the cell completes its metabolic cycle, carbon dioxide (CO_2) is released as a waste product where it's then bound to hemoglobin and carried back through your lungs. When you breathe out (exhale) this carbon dioxide is released.

You may appreciate how important all these links are in your body's essential metabolism — how they must be functioning perfectly in order that your cells retain their youthful healthy integrity.

Since your heart acts as the pump for blood, it, too, is vitally concerned with your oxygen rejuvenation set-up.

HOW PHIL OVERCAME EMPHYSEMA

Emphysema is a condition where the millions of tiny air sacs in your lungs, the ones that gather oxygen when you breathe in, lose their elasticity. The thin muscular coat around each tiny sac loses its capacity to contract down to expel the air inside it. The result is that the air sacs balloon up like grapes. The air can't be expelled. You age faster and faster.

Phil, a man I know, had such a problem.

"But how could I, Doc?" he asked, when I told him what he had. "I thought that was an old man's disease."

I told Phil that it once was, but no more. That we're seeing it with more and more frequency in young people as well.

Phil had noted that things that he used to be able to do with ease, like take hikes with his kids, play ball with them or even horse around at home on the floor with them, made him severely short of breath. And it wasn't so much, Phil said, that he felt "air hungry." He just couldn't seem to get his lungs deflated after he breathed in.

In talking with Phil, two things stood out. Several male members of his family had been afflicted with emphysema and Phil was a heavy smoker. A chest X-ray confirmed what I'd heard in Phil's chest. The black color on the X-ray film where his lung fields were pointed up the trouble. A deep black color means there is trapped air which always shows as black on an X-ray.

Phil was concerned. After all, he was only forty-seven years old and had enjoyed good health up to now. Was this the beginning of the end? The start of chronic chest disease, perhaps with early death?

The first thing I did was to convince Phil that he *must quit smoking altogether.* Usually, I'm not so stringent about smoking, but emphysema is one condition where there is no compromising — no half-way measure. It's got to be cut off completely and from then on! Phil was an inveterate smoker, and had been since he was seventeen. It wasn't going to be easy. I told Phil that I've found that the best way to curtail smoking was to follow this program:

1. Begin to take weight in hand. Use that part of the reducing diet (see Appendix) freely that shows what foods may be taken in any quantity without fear of adding useless calories. They'll help stem the desire to smoke.
2. Start a modified program of physical toning. This serves two purposes. It helps overcome the nervous desire to smoke and it helps build tone back into those loose flabby air sac muscles. Phil, of course, wasn't up to hard calisthenics or jogging just yet. He started with isometrics.
3. Whenever Phil got the "urge" to smoke, he was to go either to a window or step outside right then and there and take in a dozen breathes of fresh air *as deeply as he could possibly suck the air in.* He was to stop and interrupt whatever else he might be doing at the time to perform this important health maneuver.
4. Every night before drifting off to sleep, Phil was to concentrate completely and absolutely on the phrase: "I will not smoke another cigarette. I do not want to smoke cigarettes."

One cannot, of course, alter that which is built into his heredity. But Phil found that by altering these few things in his life, he could stem emphysema.

When he stopped smoking and began to gather a little more tolerance to his isometric exercises, I started him on a special exercise I've found helpful with emphysema. It consists simply of spending five minutes three times a day blowing up balloons! I told Phil to use the thick kind of balloon — the kind that really makes you get red in the face to blow up. When he could do this comfortably after about two months, I increased the time spent with his balloon blowing until he spent fifteen minutes three times a day at it. His tolerance to exercise went up amazingly well. He progressed to calisthenics, then eventually to jogging.

Today, Phil can play hard with his kids, take hikes and run a half mile without becoming winded. Phil overcame his emphysema. Also, it transformed him into a much younger looking and acting person.

HOW ASTHMA WHEEZING WAS STOPPED

Asthma is also an abnormal condition of air sacs. Nerves, however, play a vital, if not complete, role in this vexing condition. With asthma, the air sacs are in reverse of that in emphysema. They're constricted down so that the difficulty is in getting air *in* to the lungs.

I watched a young woman named Martha do some rather striking things with what seemed to be an intractable case of asthma.

Martha was a young woman in her early twenties, married and with three young children. Her husband was a hard working carpenter whose job waxed and waned with the construction fortunes in the community in which they lived. The family had moved to the southwest in hopes that Martha might do better with her asthma, a condition she'd had since childhood.

She had taken all the medicines. She took eight pills a day, carried a nebulizer around with her wherever she went, and still had periodic attacks of choking, wheezing air hunger and the rest. During these episodes, she required shots of adrenalin, cortisone or both to terminate her severe asthmatic attacks. Aging looks and mannerisms became almost a daily routine with her.

When I got to know Martha a bit better, and had answered several calls at all times of the day and night with these attacks, I began to tumble to the fact that she rather resented the idea that her husband wasn't able to supply her with the things she liked and wanted for her children. She wasn't actually angry at him, just unhappy with the general situation. Then it happened. Martha caught a cold, began to have one attack of asthma after another and finally developed an obstruction in the main breathing tube to the middle part of her right lung.

This catastrophe required the immediate services of a chest specialist who inserted an instrument called a bronchoscope into the blocked-off breathing tube in order to prevent disaster. Martha finally recovered completely, but it made me wonder what I should be doing with this young woman to prevent her from becoming a lung cripple. (It wouldn't take much more of this kind of episode to do the job!)

I asked Martha if she would like to go to work. She looked at me as though I were "some kind of nut" for a minute, then replied, "Yes. I'd like it very much. You know," she volunteered, "I used to be an electric motor winder, and a good one, too!"

When Martha found a job (good motor winders are hard to find, apparently) she completely got over her asthma. She was able to stop all her medicines including the nebulizer, has no special trouble with ordinary colds and her chest hasn't felt tight since. That was four years ago. A good record, and a case in point, of nerves being behind this uncomfortable, unrelenting condition.

POLLUTION NOT ALWAYS OUTDOORS

There are many ways that you can pollute the air you're breathing. And it isn't always in the great outdoors as one might be tempted to believe with all the ballyhoo given the problem in news media these days.

Norbert's case illustrates what I mean. It seems Norbert began to notice his chest trouble about six months before he came to see me about it. He said he first noticed a dry, hacking cough from time to time that gradually became more frequent as well as more nerve-racking. Often, he would cough so hard and so often, that he'd gag and vomit. Then he'd feel better. He also noticed his chest often felt "tight" and constricted as though gripped in a vice.

Norbert was in his thirties, smoked a pipe and was in apparent excellent health. In checking him over, including chest X-rays, I could find not a trace of obvious trouble. I suspected allergies. A battery of the usual skin tests were negative. I suspected a nervous condition, but an exhaustive talk with Norbert failed to turn up probable causes for such. Meanwhile, he became worse. He was weakening from his caughing spasms. A broncho-scope examination (where the breathing tubes can be seen) revealed only a red breathing tree lining.

Finally, the clue came. It seems that Norbert had just changed jobs in the plant where he worked. He was transferred to an area where newsprint and inks were used. A little testing revealed Norbert was highly sensitive to printer's ink. When he was removed from this area, his chest symptoms cleared up im-mediately!

Yes, your environment can surely age your breathing system. Don't underestimate it when looking around for reasons for your chest discomfort, whatever it may be.

AVOIDING COPD

COPD is the abbreviation for chronic pulmonary obstructive disease. We are seeing it more and more these days. The term COPD is simply a general name for anything that causes lungs to fail to work properly. The three states we've already dis-cussed, emphysema, asthma, and chronic irritants, are examples of COPD. The following program will enable you to avoid this crippler of lungs:

1. If you smoke and you're noticing any sign of lung trouble, including shortness of breath, *stop smoking.* If you smoke and haven't had lung or chest symptoms, cut smoking in half today, and by three-fourths within the next year. You'll feel better and avoid COPD.

2. Cut your alcohol intake in half, regardless of the amount you use at present. It hasn't been scientifically accepted, but I've noticed that of the many alcoholics I've examined, fully 80% or more of them have manifestations of COPD.

3. If you work in a factory, or around any material that others you know have had trouble with, have the industrial physician at the place do a simple ventilation test for you at least every year. This is done simply by exhaling force-fully into a standard measuring device that records the amount of air in your lungs. If there is a decrease in your air capacity, look for trouble with COPD.

4. Every day of your life, interrupt whatever you're doing, go to the window or outdoors and take in a dozen or more forced inspirations and expirations (breathing in and out), holding your breath as long as you can with both phases). This is your youth cocktail.

5. Learn to increase your own lung capacity by starting diaphragmatic breathing. This means using your diaphragm muscle to suck in the air before you start to expand your chest. You should learn to do both abdominal and chest breathing, but the diaphragm part of breathing is usually neglected.

6. As part of your youth toning routine, take up jogging, swimming and/or one of the running games like tennis. These activities put needed pressure on your lungs.

7. Make a point *not* to make your house air-tight, especially in winter. You need fresh air while you sleep no matter how cold it is outside.

HOW TO PREVENT PREMATURE AGING OF YOUR HEART

When the muscle fibers of your heart are stretched beyond their ability to contract efficiently, heart failure, often called cardiac decompensation, occurs. This usually happens on the left side of the heart — the side that pumps the blood returned to it from your lungs to all the rest of your body. One thing that causes a failing heart we've discussed already — high blood pressure. Being too heavy is a common cause of both heart failure and high blood pressure. Good reasons to avoid flab!

Sometimes heart failure is brought on simply by overexertion — doing much more physical effort than anyone could reasonably be expected to do.

Robby, a lean, athletic looking young man of only twenty, is such an example. He ventured to the Colorado Rockies one summer on vacation. Being from the East, he was used to the way things are at sea level, and had never been sick in his life. On the second day after his arrival in Denver, Robby and a friend decided to try their hand at mountain climbing, a sport neither had attempted before.

The friend pooped out and had to stop about a third of the way up the mountain they'd selected. Robby was also tired, but was determined to complete the climb all the way to the top. Before reaching the summit, Robby collapsed. His friend called for help and a special rescue team loaded Robby onto a stretcher, carried him down off the mountain and delivered him to the emergency room of a hospital where I first saw him.

Robby had suffered acute cardiac failure (decompensation, it's often called). His lips and cheeks had a definite bluish hue to them; his breathing was rapid, labored and shallow. His heart rate was twice normal and his ankles were swollen from the foot to half way up his legs on both sides.

Robby was lucky. He recovered in a couple of days and appeared as good as new. He might have died from his stubborn determination to reach the top. It pays to condition yourself to altitude before any such strenuous activity is undertaken. It also pays to pick a small hill to climb, not the highest peak in the state!

A STRONG HEART IS A YOUNG HEART AT ANY AGE

The following will guide you in avoiding the pitfalls of heart failure:

1. Control that weight! Ideal weight is the only thing you should settle for.
2. Start your physical toning routines now! Not next week or next month. Your heart gets a bonus through exercise no matter what group of muscles you're working on at the time — heart muscle gets stronger with any exercise!
3. If you're out of physical shape, take easy exercise routines at the beginning. If you have already had heart trouble, check with your doctor before starting anything vigorous — he can tell you the limits you can meet safely. You may be able to exceed these limits after regaining tone, ideal weight and good health.
4. After thirty, reduce salt intake three-fourths. Add salt to your diet only if you lose an especially large amount as in working in the heat and sun, during vigorous exercise or

any other unusual sweating. Salt seems to predispose in some people to heart failure. After forty-five years, depend on the natural salt content of foods for *all* your salt. Don't add it at all to foods or cooking.

5. Check with your doctor for unusual chest pain, irregularities in heart rate, swelling in extremities (feet, ankles, hands, etc.) difficult breathing in the prone position (as in lying in bed at night). Once corrected, such conditions will adapt themselves to your youth-building with proper precautions.

6. Learn to observe the red lining in your lower eyelids and the creases in the palms of your hands. The depth of redness in these areas is a good indication of the iron content of your blood. If you need iron — in other words, are anemic — have it corrected by your doctor. *Then* start youth-building. Lean meat, vegetables, raisins and wheat germ are good sources of natural iron. Use them often in your diet.

BREATHLESS FAT

I've seen many an air-starved person, but perhaps the most striking example was the case of Wendy, a forty-three year old lady who waddled into my office one day to tell me of this breathing problem she had.

Wendy was about five feet three inches tall and weighed 267 pounds! She was a living fat factory. She'd been around to "all the doctors and specialists" without results and her breathing was becoming worse. As she sat on the table, she talked in gasps and breathed like an old fashioned steam engine. Her lips were rather bluish and her face an ashen color.

One specialist, she said, had told her she had Dercum's disease. This is a very unusual and rare disease in which there are painful inflammatory changes going on in the thick rolls of fat hanging down from the chest, abdomen and backside. It is quite uncomfortable and it is not too clear what causes it. It *never* occurs, however, in a lean person.

She had taken this diagnosis with great relief. It was comforting to Wendy to have "something to lean on" — an excuse for her obesity problem. Trouble was, she didn't have Dercum's disease at all. She had just collected fat on her body in enough quantities to cause serious breathing problems.

And how can this occur? Simple! When your body stores fat, it begins to deposit it in areas of least resistance on your frame. First, the abdomen gets its share. Then the extremities. And finally, the fat has nowhere else to go but beneath your skin between it and the muscle layers.

Wendy had even progressed beyond this point! It was piling up inside her abdomen again. It had piled up so much in fact, that it was literally pushing everything out and up. When it began to push up her diaphragm, (these, remember, are the muscles that pump air in and out of your lungs and that separate your chest cavity from your abdomen), she couldn't make them work against all this fat — her flab was literally cutting off her air! When she would lay down, her breathing became more difficult, the tremendous fat deposits pushing upward by gravity in the lying down position. She had learned some time ago that she could never lay flat — if she did, she would actually undergo a kind of suffocation!

Wendy really had a tough dilemma, but she eventually licked it. And she did it simply by losing weight. I told her that if she didn't, she would probably not be around to complain about her discomfort in another year. We then went around about the usual "pills" to reduce, and about thyroid trouble and a host of other glandular disturbances. Tests on Wendy proved that her glands were not at fault. She wasn't convinced. She decided next to go to the Mayo Clinic since, as she put it, "she wasn't getting anywhere locally." So to Mayo's she went. There, she was worked up from stem to stern, given another complete physical examination and had enough blood drawn for laboratory tests to fill a quart bottle. The results were the same: Normal. The wise specialists told her to return home and get her breathing apparutus restored to normal before it was too late.

Wendy finally decided to follow through with a strict diet. She had to be hospitalized at first, so severe was her problem. She was kept on only 600 calories a day while there. A security system was set up around her room to insure that no one could sneak in food or drink, a trick she had successfully tried before. The scales succeeded in convincing Wendy that if you eat less than your body actually needs to function, it has to burn up stores of fat as a source of energy. Her weight dropped. She became a believer.

A few days of sedation were necessary; Wendy was a compulsive eater — she stuffed in food without realizing it.

Then she learned to control her mind. She was able to reduce her hunger pangs through autosuggestion and control of her nerves. It wasn't necessary to go into *why* she was nervous — the important thing to Wendy at the time was that her nervousness was driving her into an early grave. As her weight peeled off, Wendy began to become physically active again, something she had completely stopped in putting on her excess flesh. She soon found that when her tremendous abdomen began to shrink, she could do more and more exercises without running so much out of breath that it took twenty-five minutes to recover it.

Because her diaphragm muscles were weakened, I started Wendy out on diaphragm isometrics. I instructed her to do the following not less than three times daily for ten minute periods:

1. Draw air into her lungs as deeply as she could possibly make her diaphragm do so. Even to the point of discomfort. To hold this "air in" cycle as long as she could.
2. Then let the air out, forcing the last little bit out even after she felt she had breathed out as much air as there could possibly be in her lungs. To hold this cycle as long as she could before taking in another breath.
3. After five such cycles, she was to make her diaphragm move up and down without actually taking in or letting out air. This was done in a standing position, forcing the abdomen to "pooch out" as far as possible, then drawing it in again deeply enough to expand her chest. This motion moves the diaphragm vigorously and you can make them continue to do so without actually sucking in or blowing out air.
4. Later, when Wendy had dropped almost eighty pounds of weight, I started her on jogging in place, jogging outdoors, and on long walking hikes. This increased her "wind." She stopped smoking. This, in itself, had a salutary effect on her breathing capacity.

5. When she came down another thirty pounds in weight, I started her on more vigorous calisthenics. She began push-ups, sit-ups, scissor kicks, and others. The more she did of this, the better she began to breathe.

Today, Wendy weighs 126 pounds. Not quite ideal, but so much improved over the beginning that I didn't have the heart to insist she get completely down to ideal. She hasn't had a day of breathlessness in more than two years, and remains in excellent physical condition through daily physical conditioning. She looks about fifteen years younger than she did the day she steamed into my office. She probably added thirty-five years of normal, healthful life to her total span over that day!

THE MORE ENERGY, THE MORE OXYGEN

When you first start your exercise toning routines, you'll notice how "winded" you are. This is because when you ask these tired weak cells to start perking again — to start using and burning up more energy in response to your conditioning program — the two things they need is sugar and oxygen. The sugar, your body supplies, either in the form of what you've eaten that same day or what you've stored as fat. What your body can't supply is oxygen. You've got to breathe that in.

Recently, a man who had started his toning routines told me he couldn't understand why he seemed to be getting more tired and lethargic as his toning program continued. He'd been at it for about three months and had immediately noticed a change for the better. He increased his exercising time correspondingly — but now, he was "going downhill."

When I began to question him about his exercising — what he was doing, how he was doing it and where — it became evident that he was exercising in his rather small bedroom. It was winter, the climate had been cold, and his house was extremely well built, tightly put together and he had an over-size furnace to insure maximum comfort during the cold snaps.

The trouble here was that everything in this man's house was too tight, and his furnace too effective. He simply wasn't allowing enough oxygen to get into his small bedroom to keep up with his increased demand! Also, his furnace was using up a goodly supply of oxygen in burning the gas that produced his heat.

The answer proved surprisingly simple: all he had to do was to open his window and let some of that fresh oxygen in during his exercising times — thoroughly air out the room, some minutes before exercising, and for a time afterward to insure that oxygen used up by his increased demand was replaced. He has had no problems since.

LUNG DAMAGE CAN SHUT OFF AIR

There are some processes that the human lungs are afflicted with that can impair air supply. We've discussed some of them. They can't all be avoided, but most of them can with careful attention.

I met a woman of fifty who had come to the desert southwest hoping to improve what had become a chronic breathing problem for her. The desert didn't help, though she probably breathed a little easier since the desert was located at sea level and her home was located at three thousand feet altitude.

Molly had suffered a bout of what is called bronchiectasis some five years ago. This disease is caused by a number of things, but the end result is the same: "stopping up" of one or more of the smaller breathing tubes to a section of lung. When this "stoppage" is complete, the lung tissue to which the breathing tube runs collapses and scars down. When this happens, that portion of the lung can no longer assist the body in its oxygen supply — there simply isn't any way for air to get in or out of this particular section. It simply withers away.

Nature is usually kind to us humans. If a part of what we must have to survive becomes diseased, the rest — the healthy parts — are usually able to take over and do a good job. Not so, however, in Molly's case. Nature had played a cruel trick on her breathing apparatus. The rather large section of lung involved with her bronchiectasis was only partially closed — not completely. The air could get into the section of lung, but couldn't get back out — Nature had inadvertently created a kind of "ball-valve" effect. A large part of the air she breathed was rendered completely useless.

The result was that Molly was having increasing difficulty with just ordinary breathing, and even mild exercise, such as walking any significant distance, was absolutely out of the question.

Happily, for Molly, there are cures for even this very vexing problem. A surgeon was able to apply his skill to the diseased part of Molly's lung — remove it entirely so that her vital oxygen would no longer get shunted into this useless section and trapped. When she recovered in a few weeks from her surgery, Molly was a new person — literally and figuratively. She gradually built herself to the point where she could tolerate a few calisthenics and isometrics every day. She could walk as far as she wanted without running dangerously short of air, as was formerly the case. She regained about twenty youthful years by having her breathing power brought back from ill health.

TAKE CARE OF THE LRI

The term LRI stands for Lower Respiratory Infection. It is in distinction to the URI — jargon for Upper Respiratory Infection. Respiratory infections can be caused by viruses or bacteria — usually the former. When you get a head cold, that's a URI. When it gets down into your chest, then it's an LRI.

LRI's deserve special attention because of their sheer numbers — most people have such a go-round every year or two. Some more often, some less, but we all, it seems, must suffer the ravages of the "flu" or "grippe" at one time or another.

Since LRI's involve your breathing, it's important to recall some things about them when they occur. The following table will help in this regard:

1. When you start to hack or cough, and your chest feels tight, you have an LRI. Baby it along until it is over. If a fever comes along with it, see your doctor.
2. If the phlegm you cough up takes on a yellow or green color, bacterial infection has probably entered the picture even if "a cold" started the LRI to begin with. See your doctor if this occurs.
3. DO NOT pursue vigorous exercise routines during an LRI. The inflamed membranes lining your breathing tubes will

just react to the further inflammation caused by the increased air forced down them. Reduce your routines to just isometrics that don't "wind" you so much. Stop before you start to cough and hack and have chest pain.

4. Get plenty of extra rest and don't sleep with chilly night air blowing on you. This is fine when you're well, but NOT when you have an LRI. Don't go outside at night with a cough unless you really have to.

5. A good home remedy for LRI's is to get hold of an old sauce pan, fill it about a fifth full of water and stir in some compound tincture of benzoin, a solution you can pick up in your corner drugstore. Heat this mixture on a stove, lean over the vapors as they come off and slowly and deeply inhale them for twenty or thirty minutes, three or four times daily.

6. If you have trouble breathing even while resting in bed or on a chair, consult your doctor without further delay. Pneumonia can start with an LRI.

YOUNG LUNGS REQUIRE EFFORT

The time to start restoring vitality to your breathing apparatus is NOW! The better the lungs and heart going into mid-life, the better they will perform for the rest of your life. This doesn't mean you can't improve things if you've let them slip to this point. It means, in a word, that an ounce of prevention is worth a pound of cure.

Whatever you do to help your lungs along, you'll get the bonus of helping your heart stay in youthful tone as well. Recall, the exercising routine designed to tone up specific muscles as well as automatically make your air sacs expand and contract to stay flexible. The routine also stirs up heart muscle to even more vigorous tone and strength as well, and, as you have seen, helps prevent damage to the blood vessels that supply the heart and lung tissues with blood.

CHAPTER SUMMARY

1. Dynamic breathing helps you stay young. This means good heart muscle tone, good lung air sac tone and adequate fresh air.

2. Emphysema and asthma are agers of lungs. You can avoid both of them and if they do appear, you can build your youth program around them provided you follow the rules in strengthening your air sacs.

3. You can reduce the total effect of air pollution by insuring your own private pollution is kept to a minimum.

4. COPD can be avoided. You will retain a young breathing system by learning to avoid known factors that can start COPD.

5. A strong heart is a young heart. Your youth program can keep your heart strong and avoid the chance of heart failure.

6. The oxygen carrying capacity of your blood is linked to its iron content. Anemia (iron-poor blood) can be corrected and prevented.

10

How to Keep Youthful Lustre in Your Skin, Hair, and Teeth

In taking steps to properly care for your outer covering (your hide, in other words), you can retard aging and keep that youthful look. I want to discuss with you how this is done in this Chapter.

Among the natural aging processes in skin is the adolescent condition known as acne. Almost everyone goes through some acne in their life. Some have it worse than others. I want you to learn how to prevent the severe disfiguring type and what you can do if you've already gone through it.

Skin wrinkles age your appearance tremendously. I want to talk about what to do in preventing wrinkles and how to smooth them out once they appear. The same applies to sagging jowls, bags beneath your eyes and leathery skin. I want to show you how to deal with all of these aging conditions.

Hair "makes" both man and woman. It's often the first thing people look at when they meet you. I want you to learn how to keep your hair youthful and vital, and what to do about preventing baldness.

Of all your natural assets, your teeth certainly rank among the most important. Properly cared for, there is no reason they shouldn't last you a life time. I want to discuss proper care in this section.

Of course, the problem of water fluoridation, dentures and tooth paste always arise in such a discussion. I'll discuss these topics as well.

HOW TO MAKE YOUR YOUTH MIRROR REFLECT THE REAL YOU

When you look in a mirror, what do you see first? You see your face. The same thing is true when you're in public or when you're introduced to someone — the first thing they see is your face. And, right or wrong, they often judge you on the appearance of what they see in that face.

It makes good sense to keep your face looking as young as you can. As long as you're at it, why not do the same with all your body's outer covering. It will pay dividends in a more youthful appearance, and in your health in general.

Ever notice the really big difference in the appearance of an older person? Often, it's not his bent fragile looking physique or his wobbly gait. It's the sallow, lustreless appearance of a wrinkled skin. It's the sparse, thin brittle hair, and the absence of teeth altogether, or perhaps the awkward thrust of his jaw with either a single upper or lower plate without its second member present. If a person sees such a picture in the mirror everytime he looks in one, soon the mental image of aging becomes fixed. And believe me, it's very difficult to get out of such an aging rut.

It's amazing what you can do to improve such an image. It starts, of course, with prevention and runs the gamut of treatment to do away with the blemishes of age.

HOW TO DO AWAY WITH ACNE

Very often the ravages of facial acne extend well beyond the adolescent period during which it starts. Many people must suffer through it in their twenties, thirties and into mid-life. The blemishes, of course, aren't themselves serious or life threatening — they just look disgusting. And whether we admit it or not, whenever we look at such a face, we automatically avoid looking at it again. The same is true of a face that has struggled with acne and lost the battle — the deep pock-marked scars have left their aging legacy.

WHAT MEL DID ABOUT HIS UGLY ACNE

A man I know named Mel was in such a bind with his face. Already twenty-eight, his face was ravaged by large cystic blobs of acne lesions. Just when he thought he had them under control, a new batch would break out, become infected and form pustules. Soon, the lesions started breaking out on his chest and shoulders and soon extended to his back. Mel was miserable. He was embarrassed to appear in public. He was aging prematurely.

Mel, I soon learned when I examined him, was one of "the oily ones." This means that his skin was naturally quite oily. Such is true of many skins, and the condition is always accentuated by the onset of growth spurts such as occurs in adolescence.

Here is what I had Mel do:

1. Shampoo hair twice a week. Use plain bath soap for the first rinse, use special seborrhea shampoo for second rinse: Sebulex or Fostex brand or equivalent; either can be purchased in a drug store without a prescription.
2. Wash face, neck, shoulders and back three times a day. Use ivory soap at first two washings; Fostex cake soap for third, same formula as Fostex cream above.
3. No squeezing of infected or red acne lesions. Use sterilized needle to pierce pimple head; wash out "core" with warm water.
4. Special acne diet. This diet appears in the Appendix at the end of the book.
5. Shave with electric razor. Keep hair trimmed reasonably short.

With this routine, Mel's acne cleared up quite well. I had to start him for a short time on low doses of an antibiotic because of the widespread infection, but he was able to stop this drug after about three weeks.

The Basic Acne Program

The shampooing routine is important. This is because seborrhea (dandruff) flakes from an oily scalp fall onto the forehead and face, causing irritation and blackheads to form. This, in turn, makes acne worse. Blackheads should be dealt with as follows:

1. Thorough warm water soak with washcloths at night.
2. When pores in skin open from warm soak, gently remove blackhead from pore with blackhead extractor (obtainable in most good drug stores).

3. Take small area of face — remove three or four of
largest from this area only. Then rest this area and do
same with another small area the next night.
4. *Never* squeeze blackheads. It only makes things worse.

Warmth opens pores in your skin — cold closes them. Blackheads are in the bottom of pores — to get them out, pores
have to be opened first. Most people, Mel included, try to
remove too many blackheads at "one sitting" and are too
rough on the skin when they do it. I had to convince Mel this
was so by letting him do too much (in his zeal to rid himself
of the condition). Soon, Mel had large tender red areas of
infection on his face in spite of precautions. When he stopped
trying to do *too much,* this condition stopped.

It's tempting to squeeze pustules and blackheads. Besides,
you can "see the white core come out" when you do. This is
not the best method, however. The best method is to use the
blackhead extractor — a small tool with a spoon-shaped end
with a small hole in the middle of the spoon — the blackhead is centered beneath this hole and gentle downward pressure
removes the blackhead, easily and non-traumatically.

In time, Mel was able to reduce this routine to once every
other night or less. He no longer fears the public or what people
will think when he meets them — his acne problem is under
complete control. He found youthful skin once again.

WHEN SCARS ARE LEFT

Mel was fortunate that his face cleared without much scarring or pock-marking. I've seen plenty of faces that haven't.
When this unfortunate state of affairs happens there are two
alternatives: Dermabrasion, and special make-up techniques.
Dermabrasion by a skin specialist can help some pock-marked
faces tremendously. In those that can't be helped with this
technique, dermatologists (skin specialists) can resort to make-
up techniques that can completely mask the scarring and pocks.

At any rate, there are *no* other local treatments with expensive
creams, unctions, corrosives (chemicals that eat away the skin)
that will do anything but make matters worse. Such cases require
specialists that know what they're doing.

HOW TO AVOID A FACE LIFT JOB

I've lost count of the number of Ediths I've seen. She represents a peculiar problem of someone who looks twenty-five, if you judge only her figure and muscle tone, but looks fifty if you judge her face and the condition of her skin.

Edith was actually thirty-three. She lamented, "Doctor, what can I do? My face is withering away!" And she was right. The skin on her face was tough, leathery and full of wrinkles. She had bags beneath her eyes and a double chin.

In talking with Edith, I learned some things that are quite typical of her problem. First, Edith was a sun worshipper — she spent all her free time basking in the sun. She went to the beach frequently, she took sun baths on the patio at home and used a sun lamp all through the winter months!

Sunlight is fine — provided you respect it. Edith hadn't learned to respect the sun and what it can do used to excess. Oh, sure, Edith always had a fine tan. Winter or spring, Edith looked just as though she'd returned from two months in the Carribean. But she'd overdone it. She'd forgotten to use adequate sun screening *before* exposure. And she'd forgotten that when oils are cooked out of the skin, they must be replaced or the skin will dry up — permanently.

In addition to all this, Edith had two small areas on her forehead and on one cheek that were angry looking and beginning to form sores in their centers that just wouldn't heal up.

As I suspected, Edith had two skin cancers on her face. Fortunately, they were caught early and removed by a dermatologist before they had spread. In fact, Edith's skin covered the defects left by the surgical removal so well that the spots couldn't be seen from more than a foot away. I put Edith on the following routine:

1. Facial Isometrics. I've talked about these before and there is a list of them in the appendix at the end of the book.
2. Tender loving care of the skin. This included washing no more than once a day and with a completely bland soap such as Ivory. It also included *avoiding the sun altogether!* This doesn't mean Edith had to become a

household recluse for the rest of her life. It did mean that she must use an effective sun screen lotion or oil whenever she would be exposed to the sun. It also included a nightly facial: massage of the face with her finger tips using a soothing, oil-restoring lotion or cream such as Nivea (no prescription necessary) in generous quantities. It excluded all the cosmetics, facial mud and such items as women seem to enjoy putting on their faces.

3. The addition of vitamins A and C to her dietary supplement. I'll discuss the use of vitamins later in the book.

It took some time for the brown sun-tanned skin to fade away and become normal appearing again, But Edith won out — she reduced the number of wrinkles, reduced the fat pads beneath her skin and reversed the leather effect after diligence and patience. She has had no further skin cancers and has taken fifteen years off the appearance of her face.

COPING WITH THE LOOSE SKIN SYNDROME

Nothing can age the skin quite so much as the drooping jowl situation or the loose blobs of skin that hang down from various portions of the face. I've heard many people complain that this was the main reason they "hated to go on any weight losing routine." They feared their skin would hang down in aprons from their bodies, especially from their faces. This can happen, but is quite unlikely *if you also pay attention to muscle toning with weight reduction.*

The skin in your face is much like skin anywhere else. It contains oil glands, sweat glands and an underlying layer of elastic tissue that keeps it resilient and firm. Given the proper weight losing routine and the proper muscle toning along with it, there is no reason why your facial skin need droop and sag any more than anyplace else. What is often forgotten is that the skin on your face is stretched over muscles just like the skin on your chest, abdomen, legs and arms. If these muscles are toned just as faithfully and thoroughly as you are now doing with the rest of your body, your facial skin will remain smooth, firm and flexible.

**Treatment for "Bags" Beneath
the Eyes**

I recall a patient named Melissa who complained of bags beneath her eyes and a double chin that drooped so much that it gave her the appearance of a goat. Bags beneath the eyes are usually accentuated by dark circles below the lower eyelid. This can be caused by a number of things including chronic ill-health or lack of physical vitality for any reason. When muscle toning, diet and skin care were started on Melissa, the first thing to disappear was her double chin. One of the things that helped this along was an exercise she developed herself consisting of taking a small rubber ball and, holding it beneath her chin, rolling it in circles and back and forth across the dining room table three or four times a day, for five or ten minutes. She literally pulled her chin in by toning up the flat muscle that covers most of the front part of the neck. When the muscle was toned, the flab that collected over it disappeared, and the double chin along with it.

In Melissa's case, I had her expose her face cautiously to sunlight with her glasses removed. She was, of course, careful to use sun screening lotion in this process. The gradual mild tanning of the skin beneath her eyes eliminated the dark rings that stood out so prominently before. In addition to this, Melissa toned up the muscles that surround the eyelids as well as the eyelids themselves. This smoothed out the bags and they've been gone since. She removed about fifteen years from her face with this very simple routine. A routine that you can and should follow and which should be done every day just as faithfully as the ones you're using for your other muscles.

HOW TO KEEP HAIR YOUTHFUL LOOKING

Hair has become a glamour symbol with both men and women. Naturally, when it begins to deteriorate or fall out, you're concerned. Men and women have their own peculiar problems with prematurely aging hair. Let's look at them under separate headings.

MEN'S HAIR CARE

In general there are two kinds of baldness or loss of hair that afflict men. One is hereditary and one is acquired. I've said before that one cannot pick the type and characteristics of his heredity — he is born with them and that's that. If baldness has occurred in a number of the male members of a given family tree, one can look for it to occur with fair certainty. And all the mysterious hair growing treatments and lotions will be to no avail whatsoever.

The acquired type is a different story, however. Acquired means that something you're doing or have already done is causing your hair to fall out. In this kind of baldness, the areas involved are usually scattered and in well-localized parts of your scalp. This kind of trouble gives the appearance of your hair thinning out in a number of different spots. The kind of hereditary baldness I mentioned usually isn't like this, but rather gives the appearance of widespread loss of hair, typically on the top and sides of the scalp with a "fringe" of hair around the ears, the nape of the neck and the sideburn areas. The rest of the scalp is usually utterly devoid of hair and no amount of therapy will restore it permanently.

The following are points to remember in avoiding the acquired type of hair loss:

1. Men overwash their hair. Once a week is plenty. Ordinary liquid green soap is all you need to do the job, and two rinses is usually all it takes.
2. When you remove the oil from your hair after a shampooing, it's well to replace it. Hair preparations that are mostly oil and/or lubricants are best for this. The various sprays and other unctions that "smell good" and give that "manly" look to your hair are too drying and will break down the protein structure of your hair in the long run. Just plain vigorous massage of your scalp with fingers and a little lubrication will do the best in restoring vigor to your hair.
3. Anything that you use on hair to alter its color will harm hair in the long run. Accept the color you were born with and don't be dismayed by graying — it looks dignified.

The Balding Problem

I recall seeing a man named Ted who complained of this "area balding" problem. His family tree had nothing to indicate that heredity played a part in it. And his problem began just about two years ago at the age of thirty-eight. This two years of hair loss added about ten years to Ted's appearance. He was at a loss to explain it.

In talking things over with Ted, it became apparent that one of the main reasons for his particular hair loss was that he used the same soap to shampoo with that he used to "deodorize" his body with. And he always washed his hair during his daily shower. In addition, he used a spray hair dressing containing a large percentage of alcohol, which thoroughly dried his hair. In fact it dried so much that it began to wither up and fall out. All he had to do to stop this vexing state of affairs was to allow the natural oils to return to his hair. In three months he was rid of his problem, and replaced those ten years to his physical appearance.

WOMEN'S HAIR CARE

Fraying on the ends, gobs of hair falling out when combed and dry hair are the common complaints women have with their hair. They don't suffer from baldness with the frequency that men do, but it does occasionally occur. There are a number of metabolic (systemic) causes frequently offered for such conditions, however, they occur much less often than supposed. More often, problem hair in women occurs as a result of using far too many sprays, lotions, setting chemicals, wave-sets, etc., than is compatible with young vibrant hair.

As I've mentioned already, human hair is composed of a particular kind of protein fiber — just like the wool in the suit or coat you may be wearing. Anything that dries this protein excessively will cause it to fray at the ends, frazzle along the shaft and even fall out. This is also why wool clothing eventually succumbs to repeated dry cleaning.

Woman should remember the following in retaining youthful hair:

1. Wave set and spray conditioners do 80 percent of all the damage done to your hair. They all contain chemicals that cause protein to come apart — sooner or later so will your hair if you overdo these chemicals. Remember, your hair is always more vulnerable after it's shampooed — the protective oils have been removed leaving the hair vulnerable to the chemicals applied to it.

2. Tints and dyes cause the remaining 20 percent of your hair problems. These chemicals, too, contain drying agents, but more important, they contain slowly acting chemicals which, over time, can dissolve away the protein that makes up hair. They also tend to straighten out what natural curl or wave may be present and will leave your hair stringy and straggly over the long haul.

3. The longer hair grows, the more difficult its maintenance becomes. It's easier on you and your hair will stay more vigorous and healthy if you aim toward the shorter styles.

HOW TO KEEP "YOUNG" TEETH

I'm appalled at the number of young people I see in my office every day who have already lost most of their teeth and are well on their way to making it 100 percent. I can't imagine why people neglect the youthfulness that could be theirs if they'd only expend a little effort on their teeth.

People wonder why their teeth continue to rot from their mouths in this day and age of super toothpastes and even more super nutrition. I think basically people have the wrong idea about mouth care.

A young mouth does not come from brushing your teeth! It does come from brushing and cleaning your *gums!* Given a normal set of teeth, strongly enameled and solidly grounded in their jawbone ridges, they'll do fine *if the gums around them are kept in youthful condition.*

Cavities don't start in teeth. They start as decay and rot in and between gum ridges. The most important tool, therefore, in keeping your teeth youthful and healthy is not your toothpaste but your dental floss — the string-like stuff that you use to draw out the food particles from between your teeth.

Jerry, a young lad of fourteen, is typical of hundreds of thousands of such cases in this country today. His mother was convinced that he had some dread disease or metabolic disorder because he developed cavities in his teeth at the rate of about six every two or three months. He had several of his "baby" tooth pulled when he was younger and was well on his way to losing about three more when I saw him. I think neither Jerry nor his mother paid the least attention to their dentist when he was in the office innumerable times. At least, it didn't look like it. I asked about dental hygiene. "Why," said Jerry's mother, "we always use fluoride toothpaste. That's all we need to do, isn't it?"

I pointed out that while this kind of toothpaste is definitely an advance, it does just what it implies — it protects the tooth itself against cavities — it does not protect the gums.

A Tooth Care Routine

I placed Jerry on the following routine and made him vow he wouldn't vary it, even for one day:

1. Brush twice a day and after every meal. If snacks, then brush again following them as well.
2. In the evening, pull a peice of dental floss through each and every tooth interspace — between *all* the teeth, upper and lower. If he felt anything stuck bctween any teeth at any other time, then draw the floss through again whenever he felt them.
3. Before at least two brushings during every day, thoroughly scrub the teeth *and the gums* with a salt and soda mixture made at home (equal parts of each). *Concentrate on scrubbing the gums,* not the teeth. Scrub until they bleed. Keep up this vigorous scrubbing until bleeding stops, which it will when the gums are toughened up properly.

About a year later, I saw Jerry again. He had only one cavity the entire year. He was probably saved from upper and lower dentures (false teeth) at age twenty-five or thirty by applying youth-building rules to his teeth.

FLUORIDE SAVES TEETH

I won't go into all the heated arguments pro and con about fluoridated water supplies. I know it's an emotional, hotly debated subject. I just want to briefly mention Bobby, a youngster of thirteen. Bobby was from the Rocky Mountain area. He was born in 1927, a good deal before the era of water fluoridation or fluoride toothpastes. He is now forty-two years old. It seems Bobby had a grandfather who lived on a farm in Illinois. At age twelve, Bobby made regular summer sorties from his western home back to the farm to spend the holidays. Before these treks started, Bobby had the usual high number of cavities for those times, about six to eight a year. After the first two summers on the farm, his mother noticed that his two upper front teeth developed white splotches on them — mottling, as it is called. Her dentist wasn't aware of the significance of the mottling at the time, but thought it was nothing to worry about.

As the years went on, Bobby, strangely enough, didn't have one single cavity! The mottling has remained on his two front teeth, unchanged in all these years. Now, of course, we know what Bobby's problem was — the well water on the farm in Illinois where he spent his summers contained a high amount of natural fluoride. Looking in Bobby's mouth today, you can count the fillings on the fingers of one hand. Does fluoridation work? You be the judge.

CHAPTER SUMMARY

1. You can wipe away years from your body by proper care of your hide — your skin. Facial skin tolerates prolonged exposure to sun *poorly*. If you bake the oils in your skin out, replace them diligently.

2. Face lifting is rarely necessary to re-establish a youthful appearance. Careful attention to facial isometrics, general weight reduction, and to proper care of infections such as acne will re-establish youthful lustre to your face and to skin anywhere on your body.

3. Your hair reflects youth. You can preserve this reflection by protecting hair against the ravages of too many

shampoos, too much loss of natural oil, too much wave setting and permanent solution chemicals and by avoiding dyes.

4. The secret of permanently youthful teeth is in proper care of the gums and in keeping the spaces between teeth cleaned out with dental floss. Fluoridation in your water supply and toothpaste helps prevent break down of tooth enamel.

11

How to Avoid the Aging
Effects of Menopause

I'd like to discuss with both the male and the female readers in this section the subject of menopause — its myths, its truths and what to expect. I'd like to show you how easy it is to remain young, healthy and vital through this very natural time of life, the menopause.

I want to talk about so-called early menopause — what it really is and how you deal with it. I will talk about the natural sex urge and what menopause actually does to influence it.

I will show you how your body reacts to the menopause and how you can alter any adverse reaction that you may come up against. The adjustment you make to menopause is the most important factor with "the change of life," and I want you to understand how to tackle this adjustment with ease, grace and robust health.

The male aspect of menopause has been an ageless topic for discussion, mostly among people who don't really understand human abilities and disabilities any too well. I'd like to clear the air in this regard and show you exactly what happens and why.

WHAT IS MENOPAUSE?

Of all the definitions of menopause, I like this one best: Menopause is the gateway to the most productive and vital years of your life! Think of it. No longer need you women readers put up with the complete nuisance of menstruation with its pre-menstrual collection of tissue fluid, the puffiness and the irritability your frayed nerves bring. No longer need you have to cope with the messy pads or tampons and bleeding. Best of all, no longer need you fear becoming pregnant!

The reason menopause "comes along" is quite simple. Ovaries, the female sexual glands, just stop producing eggs. Without the monthly eruption of ovarian eggs, there is no menstruation. And when menstruation stops, menopause has started.

You now have the golden opportunity of your life. You can attend to all those things you've put off — without the burden on your system of losing a goodly amount of blood every month, you'll feel better, have more zip and energy and can keep up with your exercise, diet and mind control routines without interruption. You can be creative 100 percent of the time instead of just 70 percent or less. And you can now approach any problem or goal you set without the handicap of having to adjust every three or four weeks to the complex hormonal imbalance that menstruation brings. You're free!

HOW TO STAY OUT OF THE
MENOPAUSE RUT

One day Myra came to the office looking like she'd just lost her best friend. She was saddened, dejected and obviously depressed. She shuffled along as though she might be on her last leg and looked haggard and worn. After a few minutes of talking, Myra blurted out the trouble. "I think I just started menopause!" she exclaimed. "Will hormones help? How long will it take? What do I tell John?" (her husband) she asked in rapid fire order as though her very life depended on the answers. Myra was about to trip in the menopause rut. She had known her periods were slowing down and becoming lighter and further apart the past few months. She hadn't had any bleeding or spotting now for three months. And so she assumed she was automatically headed for dire straits! What was making Myra slide into this rut? A lot of malarky and wild tales from would be helpful friends, a feeling of helplessness and a bit of quite natural depression. In short, Myra was talked into her rut — preconditioned, so to speak, by what she viewed as the inexorable horror of menopause!

The first thing I did was to remind Myra of her past history. It had been completely free of serious illness, she had a fine family and a considerate husband and thirty years of potentially fruitful and happy years ahead of her as well. "But what will I do," she asked, "about all the things that go with 'the change'? Getting fat, losing my hair, turning sexless. I feel terrible already!" "You'll do essentially what you've always done, only much more efficiently and better," I replied. I told her that as far as getting fat was concerned, she could forget it completely. "Just because you've stopped menstruating," I told her, "doesn't mean you're going to put on any weight whatsoever. If you keep doing the things you know will keep your weight down. It means," I continued, "that if you watch your diet just like always and keep up your muscle toning, your weight won't change a pound." Myra wasn't convinced. I could tell by the sad look on her face.

"As far as losing your hair is concerned, you'll not be bothered by that at all unless something comes along later to cause it to happen or unless you fail to follow the guidelines for healthy hair I've already discussed with you."

I knew I was coming to the $64 question. "Sexuality has absolutely and positively nothing whatever to do with menopause," I said. "Your desires become even stronger and more satisfying because you don't have the spectre of pregnancy in the background to inhibit you any longer." Myra's face brightened up considerably. "You mean it doesn't — disappear? Doesn't die out completely?" She seemed surprised. I reassured her again that it most certainly did not. In fact, I added that I'd be surprised if her urge didn't increase!

I then pointed out that her biggest hang-up right now was the fact that she was depressed — blue and sad because she was expecting something to happen that didn't exist. I told her further, that the quickest way out of such depression was a temporary change of scenery and a strenuous program of physical activity. Myra returned to the office about six weeks later, a completely changed person. She was bright, alert and looked as trim and fit as I'd ever seen her. And all this without drugs or medicines! She'd had her change of scenery, and had her diet, physical condition and cycles under excellent control.

HOW TO DODGE EARLY MENOPAUSE

Willa, a healthy woman of thirty-six, came into the office with the flat statement that she was "going through menopause early and could she please have something for it!" On questioning her, Willa stated that "most of the women" in her family tree had "early menopause" and so naturally she was predetermined to go through it as well.

It turned out that the only reason Willa thought she was in "early menopause" was because she'd begun to notice "hot flashes." This meant menopause. I asked Willa if she'd had any changes in her menstrual pattern. No, she hadn't. Any change in the condition of the moist lining of her vagina. No, it was the same as it had always been. Any change in sex activity? "Why, yes," she said, "I've noticed that I'm just not interested anymore."

It turned out that Willa's "hot flashes" were nothing more than sweating a little more than usual with chores that involved physical exertion. This wasn't surprising in view of the fact that she'd gained fifty-five pounds over the past five years! I reminded her that being quite a bit overweight does indeed reduce sexual response and desire.

A PROGRAM FOR MAKING THE BEST OF MENOPAUSE

The point is, in Willa's case there was a hastily reached conclusion based on completely erroneous facts. I pointed out to Willa that menopause should not be entertained as a cause for symptoms unless menstrual periods have sharply diminished or stopped completely. Only then can menopause be blamed for anything. And then, I told her, there are really very few signs of it — all of which can be overcome.

I put Willa on the following routine:

1. Weight reduction. She was about sixty-five pounds overweight, having been a little over ideal weight for her frame when she started to gain excessively.
2. Physical conditioning routine. I told her there was no better substitute for getting back a youthful feeling again and throwing off false menopause than to restore tone to flabby muscles.
3. I pointed out that in her present frame of mind, she could hardly be expected to be active sexually, let alone attractive to her husband. She was to fix her hair, present herself attractively to her husband in the evening, stop feeling so sorry for herself and begin to recognize that her

husband had his problems too, but was much less able to get them off his back since he was the bread winner in the family.

A year and a half and fifty pounds later, Willa was transformed into a pert figure of a woman, attractive, well-built and in good physical tone. Her mental outlook changed completely even in the face of continual pressure from sisters, aunts and friends who had "talked" her into an early menopause. She discovered there was no such thing!

SEX AND THE MENOPAUSE

Meaning for Men

I've never seen evidence for, nor have I read any convincing work that supported the contention of a male menopause. It's hard, however, to convince people of this, to get them over the idea that at some certain critical age they may as well fold up their tents and leave home. The sex urge in men seems to be a function purely and simply of their general physical well being. At age forty, for example, men have roughly half the desire they had at twenty. At sixty, their desires are roughly a fourth that at twenty. At eighty, roughly a sixth to an eighth, and so on.

I talked with a man named Jeff who was sixty-eight. He was convinced he was losing his manliness because he'd heard that it happens to men between fifty and sixty. He couldn't understand, however, why he kept having nocturnal emmissions — wet dreams. He thought this meant he might be getting cancer of his prostate. His examination was completely negative. Of course, his prostate was a bit larger than usual — distended by secretions that hadn't been discharged because he thought his sexual days were over. When he initiated sexual contact with his wife again, his wet dreams stopped.

Meaning for Women

The age of menopause does vary from woman to woman. It generally comes on between the ages of forty-two and fifty. It is unusual for it to begin before forty or after fifty.

A woman, Lana, an intelligent and otherwise reasonable person, once argued with me for an hour or more about sex and menopause. How, she argued, could it be possible that sex urge could remain if the ovaries, the female sex glands, stopped functioning? The flaw in her argument is a common one. The ovaries *do not* stop functioning. They *do* stop ovulating. In addition, there are other sources of female hormones beside the ovaries. Both the master endocrine gland, the pituitary, and the adrenal glands contribute to estrogen formation.

Joan had become convinced that the onset of her hot flashes and drying out of the membranes in her vagina was proof positive that her ovaries had ceased their function altogether. They had *diminished* their function and, in her case, the slackening was somewhat prolonged. But they had not ceased functioning completely. Lana used an estrogen suppository for about a year to re-establish the moist condition in her vagina. After this interval, she discovered her sexual ability and interest was as high as it ever was.

ROBUST YOUTH IS POSSIBLE AFTER MENOPAUSE

There is no doubt that there are hormonal changes that occur in both men and women after the age of forty-five or so. Such changes in women are first seen in the activity of the pituitary gland — the master endocrine gland located in your brain. The chemical hormone that matures and ripens eggs in the ovaries stops being secreted. No more eggs come to blossom, hence, no menstruation. Ovaries continue to secrete estrogen, however, they do not wither away and disappear.

When the pituitary gland slows down, there is, in both men and women, a reflection of this slowing in the thyroid, the pancreas, the adrenals and the ovaries and testes (male sex glands). Notice I said *slowing* not stopping. When all these other endocrine glands slow down, naturally, some adjustments have to be made.

Consider the following in making such adjustments:

1. Slowing thyroid: this means your energy isn't burned with quite the speed as before. It means take in less carbohydrate and sugar (sources, remember, of your body's

energy) and more protein (source, remember, of muscle building). If you were on a dietary routine before age forty-five be even more strict with it now.

2. Slowing pancreas: this means less response to sudden needs or demands for energy and reduction in burning of body sugars. Review carefully the sections on diet again, and recall that the sugar cycle is directly controlled by your pancreas — get this cycle under absolute control.

3. Slowing adrenals: this means less adrenalin and regulatory hormones in your system. Learn to control your "fight or flight" response to the stress of living. Physical toning helps with this control — be even more strict with your conditioning now than before. Mind plays a vital role in your attitudes to stresses and strains. Review this section again and let nothing stand in the way of your mind's complete control.

4. Slowing sex glands: this means some diminution in sexual desire. I've already pointed out that, especially in women, this is offset by the release from sexual inhibition that inability to become pregnant brings about. Men will notice nothing in the way of sudden change — only that the desires and capabilities are simply not as strong and sustained as at age twenty.

HOW TO AVOID INVOLUTIONAL MELANCHOLIA

The term "involutional melancholia" is an old one, and, I'm afraid, a dreaded one as far as some are concerned. It means, simply, a more than usual reaction to menopause, and is applied only to women as there seems to be no counterpart in men. You can't always tell who will have this trouble and who won't, but a good idea is generally present long before this severely depressing state arrives in full force.

As a case in point, Ida, at thirty-nine, was predictable. Ida would, without much doubt, have involutional melancholia if her ways weren't changed before her menopause came along.

Ida was a completely introverted, close-mouthed, self-pitying worry wart of a person. All her life, she'd been retreating from various parts of her life until she was effectively walled off from the people and things around her. She was not psychotic. She was not a recluse or hermitess. She had formed the personality over the years, and she was a good mother and wife. Excellent at both, as a matter of fact. I was able to convince Ida to change in the following ways over a long period of time, but before menopause occurred:

1. Ida was actually a very dependent person. Her real and imagined needs in this regard were never really met. Without psychiatric intervention, Ida faced this with the help of her family — her family let her know she was important — essential — to the welfare of the family. She responded.

2. Ida had a lot of anger in her make-up, anger that was hardly ever vented but most often turned inside — on Ida herself. Such inverted anger generally creates depression from all kinds of guilt. Ida responded to physical conditioning and diet. She learned to blow off steam, so to speak, and do so in perfectly acceptable ways. She also acquired some new interests that allowed her to express her angers and hostilities so they didn't continue to "eat on her insides."

3. Ida conditioned herself to "think through" the endless chain of worries that bombarded her troubled mind all the time. When she mastered the art of examining closely the worry — looking at it logically and without the attached emotion she usually wound up with, the worry was put in perspective — whittled down to size so she didn't have to lay awake nights thinking about them.

In short, Ida simply mastered for herself many of the basic rules of youth retention we've already discussed in this book. The main trouble was that Ida waited too long before she started. It was in time, though, because she sailed through menopause without a ripple. Today, Ida is one of the happiest people I know, and she looks five years younger than her forty-six years.

MENOPAUSE: A YOUTH STEPPINGSTONE

A woman I know named Milly demonstrates the amazing transition that menopause can bring as far as youthfulness and a zest for life is concerned. Milly had been an average person all her life. She had a high school education, married young and raised a family of seven fine youngsters. She came from modest circumstances and raised her family under somewhat trying times financially, only to lose her husband when she was thirty-six.

Menopause came unusually early for Milly two years later when she had to have her uterus and ovaries removed for medical reasons. She took estrogens for about two years, then tapered off entirely.

It was as though Milly threw off heavy chains after her operation. She began to realize the profound strengths that resided in her mind. She began night school to learn typing, short-hand and business machine operation. In a year, she landed a good job with a company as an executive secretary. She completed her college degree by going to night school and successfully saw her last two children through high school. Then she helped her first two youngsters get a college education for themselves. These two, in turn, helped the rest of the kids get their college educations until all the family had college degrees.

Milly then opened her own business, an accounting firm. Small at first, then growing under her supervision and two of her sons until it is now one of the most respected in town. Today at sixty, Milly looks forty-five, feels thirty. Certainly an outstanding example of the youthfulness that can be yours following menopause.

CHAPTER SUMMARY

1. Only women experience menopause. It is the gateway to your most productive and vital years. Don't allow yourself to be influenced otherwise by those whose lives have fallen into a rut.

2. You needn't go through early menopause, nor suffer sexually during this time. Women usually desire more sex by being rid of the fears of pregnancy. Men desire about half the sex they did at the age of twenty during the time of their wife's menopause.

3. All your endocrine glands undergo adjustment at menopause. The more attention you pay to diet control, muscle

tone, mind and cycle control, the easier your adjustment will be.

4. There is no limit to your powers of youth-building, even during and after menopause.

12

How to Stay Young After Your Sixty-Fifth Birthday

Getting young at or after retirement isn't difficult. I want to talk about how you can do it in this section.

Planning for this time of your life is important. I want to discuss some items that seem to me important in this regard. Forewarned is forearmed in remaining a youthful, active, healthy person.

Marriage and the family are still important to you beyond retirement years. I want to point up how you can give a youthful cohesiveness to marriage and your family and they, in turn, will view you through different eyes by doing what you need to do.

Retirement is really a state of mind: someone's mind, unfortunately, that's occupied with other than your welfare. To solve this problem before it comes may save you a lifetime of premature aging that can be avoided easily. I want to talk about how this is done.

There are a few health needs that are peculiar to retirement years. Heading them off will allow your youthful physique and inner workings to perk along at as good a pace as ever. I want to show you how to do it with ease.

Finally, I want to explain the philosophical key that will sustain your youthful outlook throughout your entire life span.

It's so simple you'll wonder why you hadn't thought of it before.

WHAT YOU'VE GOT THAT NO ONE ELSE HAS AFTER FIFTY

I confess I get a little out of sorts when I talk to a lot of people of fifty or sixty who seem to feel their only hope with whatever they do is to hang on until they're retired. What a waste! What short-sightedness!

How Gil Recovered His Youthfulness

Gil was such a person. Gil was fifty-five and with his company for twenty-four years. He complained of being tired, nervous and out of it in general. What Gil meant to say was that he had become completely bored with what he was doing, and with life as a whole. I began to pry out of Gil what it was that really bugged him. It seems Gil started out with his company with a flash. He was a "new generation whiz kid" and really went to town. He'd worked hard at sales for a few years, then at being a supervisor for a few more. Then he landed an executive job — a minor one, but nevertheless a good one with unlimited potential. And there he'd stayed. No more zip. None of the flashy get-up-and-go for Gill. He just vegetated where he landed.

When I asked him one day why he thought his life took this turn he answered, "I don't know, I suppose I ran out of whatever it was that gave me the drive I used to have. Besides," he went on, "you have to play it cool nowadays in business — you know, don't make waves?"

I said, "No, I don't know. Did someone tell you not to 'make waves'?" Gil looked puzzled for a minute, then said, "No, I guess not, but no one has to. I've seen men higher up than I am get the axe. I'm playing it smart!"

"And suffering because of it!" I replied.

Gil was afraid. Afraid of losing his cherished rut and having to climb out. He was suffering from what I call "executive rot." But it's not at all peculiar to executives.

I talked Gil into doing just one thing after I assured him his health was excellent. I talked him into promising me he'd start the very next day looking at his company as an organism. As a living body composed of smaller essential parts all of which were working toward the good of the whole — working toward the betterment of the company, but equally important, in the process, toward the betterment of every individual in the company. I told him to start taking a close look at what others were doing — what people his age and older were contributing to the cause. I advised him to familiarize himself with the innermost workings of other departments. Burn the midnight oil if necessary, but get acquainted with other parts and other areas besides his own.

Then start to work seeing how things could be improved — made better and more efficient for all concerned.

I didn't see Gil for some months after our conversation. When I did, Gil had a bright look, a smile and a bounce in his step I hadn't noticed before. He told me that he decided to take my advice, much against his better judgement, and it worked! He said he became interested in what was going on in his own department as well as in others. He'd made suggestions that really worked and saw his own group respond to just taking an interest — a dynamic interest in what was happening. Gil, in other words, had let habit and rut take over his life. When he threw off the shackles, he opened up new vistas he hadn't been able to see before.

DOING YOUR THING — HOW TWO PERSONS DIFFERED DOING IT

I shudder when I think how many people in this country — in the world over for that matter — are devoting eight or more hours a day doing something in which they have no interest, have no special talent for, have complete boredom with and generally grow miserable while doing.

Actually, it's all a matter of preparation — preparation of body, mind and soul, if the latter plays a big part in your life. Woody is a man of seventy I know who neglected such preparation. Dean is the same age, but took care of his "homework" beforehand. The two men are as different in their retirement as day is from night.

Dean was a carpenter during his working years. He liked it. He did it well. He was in enough demand as a "finish carpenter" for new homes, he never worried about seasonal slow-downs, strikes and the like. About ten years this side of retirement, Dean started thinking about what he'd do when the time came. His wife was living and in good health, his kids were grown, married and had their own families, and Dean, himself, was in excellent physical condition. One thing he'd neglected for himself that he didn't for his kids was an education beyond high school. He decided to remedy this by enrolling in college. Not just up and quit his job — he started at night school and took one course or two at a time. He took on no more than he could handle. In the span of about eight years, Dean had enough credits to graduate with a degree. When he retired shortly before graduation, he'd become so engrossed in his studies, he decided to take up law when he retired. It took Gil about three years to acquire a law degree.

Then he made the *coup de grace*. He took a part time job consulting with the union to which he used to belong as legal adviser! He's at it today at seventy-three and going strong.

Woody, on the other hand, worked for the railroad all his life. No outside interests, no thought of retirement, no preparations. He coasted into retirement one day totally unprepared. They gave him the traditional gold watch for long and faithful service, then forgot him completely. Oh, Woody enjoyed his new freedom for a time — he hunted a little, fished and did some local traveling with his wife. But soon he became bored and frustrated, and that's when things went from bad to worse. At sixty-seven, Woody presented himself in my office one day completely irascible — his wife, complained he wouldn't take care of himself, eat right and all he wanted to do was sit in a chair on the porch and rock. Woody was deteriorating from retirement rot!

In time, and with much prodding, Woody began to move off his duff and develop an interest in his only semi-hobby before he retired — that of making model steam engines of those big work horses of the railroad that were no longer operating. In time, he was able to get engrossed in them again. Today, Woody is happier than ever since retiring, has zest for his models and is an authority who is in demand by groups interested in preserving the railroad heritage through preservation of our trains. He almost slipped into complete bondage through neglect of his golden years of life.

HOW THE JOHNSONS STAYED YOUNG
GROWING OLDER WITH THEIR FAMILY

I see a lot of people every day who complain that their parents are just withering away — they don't seem to be able to do anything or seem interested in anybody outside their own little circle of house and yard into which they've withdrawn and into which they've pulled their former world with them. Such people are simply suffering the ravages of mind and body dissolution.

They haven't kept either mind or body functioning up to par and they've forgotten about their cycles. The Johnsons, on the other hand, are people who have grown up with their family — and have stayed young in the process. Here's how they did it!

1. Instead of being the "ultimate authorities" with their kids, the Johnsons took the attitude that they had a lot to learn from their youngsters. They often consulted them about problems in and out of the family and listened when the children spoke rather than turn deaf ears "on the young whippersnappers." Consequently, the kids had a natural respect for Dad and Mom Johnson; not a lot of hostility and disappointment.

2. As the children aged, the Johnsons found they had to increase their physical tone to keep up with them. Instead of lying around the house during holidays and weekends, the family moved out and did their activities together — hiking, bike riding, swimming, shooting baskets, hunting, fishing and the like. To do this well, they found physical conditioning a necessary part of their daily routine. This in turn, toned their minds — they thought along with the children, instead of trying to act as judge and jury regarding the younger generation. There was no generation gap here simply because the Johnsons didn't let one form.

3. In the process, the Johnsons learned that they had developed a lot of outside interests in their "growing up with their children" projects. When the youngsters finished high school they enjoyed themselves doing things they liked and that kept them physically toned and mentally sharp. The children sought them out for the many problems and frustrations the big world always brings, rather than to avoid them like the plague.

4. At retirement, the Johnsons were a welcome pleasure at the homes of the children, now married and with families, rather than the "old battle axes" some parents become. They were young in heart and mind at age sixty-five because they knew no other way to be.

The Johnsons represent better than anything I know what conditioning does for you. What keeping your bodies, your minds and your cycles young and flexible can do for you. All this is built, of course, on the substance of the first eleven sections of this book. If the first five sections seem somewhat cloudy or misty in your mind at this point, I urge you to review them again. And resolve today to start youth-building for tomorrow!

THE MARRIAGE PARTNERSHIP
AFTER SIXTY-FIVE

The young marriage is the happy one. And this applies regardless of age. How do you keep marriage young? Exactly like you keep yourself young — you work at keeping yourself in good physical shape; you work to keep your mind bright and alert; you control those cycles; you keep your organism healthy and free of disease; you think about your spouse — every day. You think about the things you can do to make the day a bit easier on him, or her, and you set about to do these things.

Bill and Carol's Case

Bill and Carol, married forty years, had the correct approach. Carol had gone to work when the children were grown and away from the house. Did Bill sit around grousing and moaning about it? Did he deride Carol for having put on the "pants in the family," as I have heard so many do? No. Instead, he gave her encouragement at every turn, realizing Carol was simply fulfilling an ambition she'd had for many years, namely, to contribute. Contribute to the family coffers as well as contribute her own talents to something useful. In Carol's case, she was an expert seamstress and held a good position as knitting and sewing instructor in the fabric department of a large department store.

Bill, on the other hand, soon retired from his job with a large plastics firm. As soon as he retired, he reactivated himself in the field of helping others. There were plenty of kids in his town, much less fortunate than his own had been. He took a job as recreation councelor for a neighborhood YMCA youth rehabilitation group — working with kids from less fortunate backgrounds. He enjoys every minute of it. He stays young because he's a youthful person — he raised his own kids as part of a family, not willy-nilly, to have a good time and to heck with the rest attitude. He kept his mind sharp and his body in good condition. At sixty-seven, Bill looks fifty-five. Carol even younger.

HOW TO PRODUCE AT SEVENTY

A couple I know named Wendell and Sally didn't think retirement communities or the rocking chair were for them at sixty-five. They decided to open a business of their own at this time. Neither one had worked a business except as an employee for somebody else. But they had good ideas and knew enough to get advice from people who knew the ropes. They prospered. Why? Because they were young people!

First, Wendell and Sally picked out a spot they wanted to live in for the remainder of their lives. They picked Canada — the Canadian Rockies, to be specific. When they decided this, they contacted the Canadian government and asked for information and details on starting a business there — what it took in the way of licenses, capital, rules and regulations regarding immigrants and so on. Within a year, they had started a thriving shop in one of Canada's most beautiful and popular national parks selling English and Canadian made woolens to tourists. They are happy, they are youthful. They are productive. And they come and go as they please, living in the southern United States in the winter, and in beautiful Canada during the summer. And the business has prospered so well, they are expanding. Very shortly, they will have to expand even more to keep up with their successful enterprise!

THE KEY IS HARMONY

Again, we see that harmony brings youthful zest and energy to life. Earlier in the book, I discussed the idea of bringing into harmony the various factors of your organism that must work together and in unison to keep efficient the machinery of life. I talked about mind-body; about spirit and about cycles and the various organs and their place in the harmony of youthful living. If this harmony is interrupted, breaks down for any reason — youth begins to fade. But there is no reason that it should. You can keep harmony, therefore youth, flowing through your organism by following the simple rules already outlined in this book.

But there is yet another area where harmony plays a part. This is the area of life, in general — how you see things from your own perspective. How you absorb the rough spots in your life. How you deal mentally with those things that come up to make you stumble and falter. In other words, your philosophy of life.

I've alluded already in the book to mental outlook — philosophy. Now is the time to come to grips with it. Now is the time to bring the wisdom of experience to play to bring youth back to your thinking. The following is the key to philosophic harmony:

1. Acceptance with grace. Everything and everybody in this world, no matter how evil or shameful some of it may be, got that way through a series of events over which few have control. Accept this, and you take a step to peace of mind that will allow your youth springs to flow with increasing vigor.

2. Entrance on new ground. You may find it quite stimulating to make routine some of the things in your life. Conditioning, mind control, cycle control and mealtimes may be a few such things. But this should not make you hold back from doing other things entirely different. Entirely out of phase, so to speak, with what has been usual or habit for you. This is what lends the spirit of adventure and gives challenge to the harmonious life — it's what adds color to your life. Try something different once in a while. You'll stay younger for it.

3. Flexibility. Often we stumble across things during the course of an otherwise normal day that seem to be just the opposite of that which we understood to be correct. Seize upon these moments. Turn them around in your mind and get to the source of them. You may find an entirely new source of pleasure and enjoyment as well as revise your thinking completely regarding something you thought "was cut and dried."

GOOD HEALTH AFTER SIXTY-FIVE

There are a few things that require more careful attention as one approaches retirement so that your organism remains healthy. The following table will be helpful in considering these:

MEN	WOMEN
1. Chest trouble. Chronic coughs and shortness of breath requires attention early. Always check it out with your doctor.	1. Lumps in the breast. Have these thoroughly checked out at their first appearance by your doctor.
2. Bowel habit change. If these habits go through a change of any sort that is not the usual for you, have your doctor look into it.	2. Abnormal bleeding. If any bleeding or unusual vaginal discharge occurs after menopause or at times after intercourse, have your doctor check it out immediately.
3. Urinary trouble. If dribbling, difficulty getting your stream started or a lot of having to get up at night to urinate occurs, don't put off having it checked.	3. Urinary trouble. If you notice progressive difficulty "holding" your urine and must immediately get to the bathroom at the first sign of urine in the bladder or face losing some before you get there, don't hesitate to go in for check and repair.

CHAPTER SUMMARY

1. You have plenty to offer yourself, your marriage, your family and your community when you pass fifty. Learn what they are and put them to use today.

2. Retirement requires some planning and preparation. In the main, the elements of youth as given in the previous eleven chapters of this book will stand you in excellent

stead in such planning. Don't neglect any of the sections in such preparation.

3. You can be an asset to your family, become reactivated after formal retirement and use or not use retirement communities as you feel the need. Look carefully before you leap into retirement.

4. Harmony of body, mind, spirit and the society in which you find yourself brings youthful, golden years. Build this harmony with care and diligence utilizing what you already know about youth to do so.

5. Some health needs should be watched for, and corrected, for efficient youth after fifty or sixty. Don't put off their repair or refurbishment in the hope they'll go away by themselves. Early correction will add youth.

13

The Art of Keeping Your Hormones at Youthful Peak at Any Age

There are many notions about hormones in the human body that are, I find in talking to people, grossly misunderstood. I want to discuss the various hormones in your body, what they do and don't do, and how you can keep them up to par.

The human endocrine system, the cluster of glands in your body that produce hormones, is a fabulously balanced and regulated system. This regulation is under some conscious control. I want you to understand how this control works and what you can do to make it better and last longer.

Many people believe that there are marked differences in the way the human female hormone system works as compared to the hormone system in the human male. There is really only one important difference between the two, and I want to talk about what this is and what women must do differently than men in keeping their hormones up to snuff. There are likewise a host of misconceptions regarding the taking of hormones by pill or shot — what such therapy will or won't do for your body's youthful state. I will clear up these questions in this section and show you what to look for in deciding what hormones to take, and when to take them.

Since the advent of "the pill," the popular use of birth control hormones are pertinent to any discussion of hormones. I will talk about these and show you what you may expect or not expect of them in your youth-building. The pill has come up for much criticism recently in the press and even on television and radio. I will clear up some of the muddy waters that some of these discussions have created.

YOUR ENDOCRINE SYSTEM

The system of glands in your body that regulate virtually every vital process that goes on in it is called the endocrine gland system. The chief of these glands is called the pituitary gland, and this small but mighty cluster of cells is located in a small bony pouch about midway in the skull at the base of your brain. Your pituitary not only controls the function of every other endocrine gland in your body, but also is the center of production of the hormone that causes growth and division of every cell in your body as well as a hormone that closely regulates the activity of your kidneys. Any wonder the pituitary is called the body's master gland?

The following table will help you to understand the functions of your various endocrine glands:

1. Pituitary: Controls all other glands in addition to growth and kidney activity.

2. Thyroid: Controls the metabolism of every cell in your body. This means the control of the rate at which cells burn the energy delivered to them.

3. Parathyroid: Controls the body's calcium levels, vital to activity of muscle cells and others.

4. Pancreas: Controls the level of vital blood sugar in your system.

5. Adrenal: Makes all the cortisone-like drugs manufactured in your body. These, in turn, regulate such vital processes as the sodium and potassium cycles discussed earlier in the book, mobilize your defenses against invasion by viruses and germs and protect your cells against stresses and strains of living.

6. Sex Glands: (ovary: female; testicle: male)
   Control the production of the egg and sperm respectively and influence the sex urge as well as hair growth, mucous membrane and muscles and bones.

The most recently discovered phenomenon regarding your endocrine system is proof that the pituitary gland, the master endocrine gland, is itself greatly influenced by a small but very potent area of your brain called the hypothalamus. This area of your brain lies just above and completely surrounds the pituitary gland. The hypothalamus area actually makes potent chemicals called neurohormones that speed up or slow down the activity of your pituitary. Your hypothalamus, in turn, is intimately bound up with the emotional control of your mind. It is often referred to, in fact, as the "emotional switch-board" of your brain.

This concept is extremely important for you to know about and understand. The reason is this: for the first time, we now know (aren't just guessing as we used to be) that emotional problems can and do indeed affect your vital body processes through the mechanism I just talked about — that is, through the hypothalamus, the pituitary and, ultimately, all your endocrine glands!

See how vitally important it is that you strive for mind control? See how you, in proceeding with youth-building, can actually influence your critical endocrine system?

HOW TO INFLUENCE YOUR ENDOCRINE GLANDS TO KEEP YOUNG

Thyroid

Grant, a thirty-eight year old man, weighing 295 pounds, standing five feet nine inches tall and looking like a moving over-stuffed sofa, came into my office stating he wanted to be put on thyroid medicine because "some of my friends told me my fat is from not enough thyroid." Grant's thyroid was *not* at fault. He had simply developed the habit of shoveling in far more calories than his normal thyroid could possibly burn as energy. The only thing that his body could do with this excess energy was to convert it to fat and store it. And Grant had enough stored for three ordinary people!

You can protect your thyroid from overwork by doing as I finally convinced Grant he should do: get his weight down through diet and physical toning.

Parathyroid

Meg, a nineteen year-old woman, complained of extreme fatigue, nervousness, irritability and weight loss. Lately, she was having severe muscle cramps on the slightest exertion and suffered from "black-outs." Meg truly believed she was dying of a dread disease. Actually, what Meg had was deficient parathyroid activity. She never drank milk, ate bread or baked goods, or got out in the sun. She was short of Vitamin D — an essential ingredient of the hormone the parathyroid glands make.

To keep your parathyroids in order: protect your skin from harm with a good sun-screening preparation (see section IX) and acquire a good, even sun tan when the seasons permit. During winter seasons, see that you drink plenty of *homogenized* skim milk. This means milk that has Vitamin D added to it. Vitamin D also is found in fish oils, cereals and grains.

Pancreas

Miles, a thirty-three year old man, complained of nervous fatigue, fainting spells, shakiness, weakness of muscles and extreme jitters. He was badly out of physical shape, drank too much liquor and his eating habits were atrocious. He had the low blood sugar syndrome — his pancreas was being over-stimulated by bad habits.

Miles stopped all his trouble by eating six meals a day, smaller than regular meals, by reducing his carbohydrate (sweets and starchy foods) intake 70 percent, limiting his booze to one or two drinks at a time, and by following the principles of mind control and physical conditioning I've already outlined in this book. He also stopped drinking black coffee, tea and cola drinks.

Adrenal

Judy, a forty-six year-old lady, was a thin, undernourished, nervous person who went to pieces at the slightest provocation. She was convinced she was chronically ill and was developing arthritis in several joints, had a propensity for hives and was sexually stifled. Judy was not suffering a dread disease, though left unattended it could have been. She was allowing her adrenal glands to wither.

When Judy got hold of her mind — convincing herself she had it inside her to whip her troubles — she solved her nutritional inadequacies and regained her weight by using more protein (meat, cheese, dairy products and pod vegetables). She regained her physical tone by daily exercise routines (twenty minutes three times a day, *every day*) and stopped over-reacting to every little thing she viewed as a setback in her life. Her adrenals resumed their natural function and she threw off the shackles of "chronic illness."

Sex Glands

Sex gland activity is highest at about twenty or twenty-one years of age. This is true of both men and women. From this time forward, sex gland activity *gradually* and *slowly* diminishes, but never stops completely as I've said before in the section on menopause.

Body vigor seems the best stimulus to sex gland activity — yet another recommendation for sound and continuing physical conditioning and mind control. Not the kind that absolutely wears you down, but the middle of the road I've discussed where some physical conditioning becomes a part of your everyday activities. Not necessarily all day, just a portion of the day. This physical activity stimulates sex glands. The stimulation of sex glands, in turn, causes the muscles and mind to be stimulated. And the circle thus produced offers you a built-in sex gland protection that all the medicines, love potions and hormone shots can't approach!

YOUTHFUL MEN VERSUS YOUTHFUL WOMEN

Women

The only significant difference in a woman's hormone constitution from that of a man is the estrogen her ovaries produce. Too many women are led to believe that with the advent of menopause, her estrogen is gone — she is chemically castrated. Nothing to it! True, estrogen production decreases moderately, but quite enough remains to keep you wholly a woman.

Susan felt inadequate as a woman when menopause stopped her menstruation at age forty-eight. She lost interest in sex, she gained weight and became depressed. Was this castration?

Absolutely not! It was a psychological frame of mind induced by poor acquaintance of the facts and a lot of hogwash from her cronies who insisted that she go through the agony they had to. When Susan overcame her depressed moodiness by mind control and got back in physical shape, she regained all the sexual vigor she had ever had and felt fifteen years younger in the process.

Men

Testosterone, the hormone produced by the testicle that makes men uniquely men, gradually diminishes over the years without the sudden diminution that women notice. Again, I reiterate, the only thing you need to do to keep the testicles healthy and producing enough hormones to maintain good and vigorous manlihood is to keep in good physical and mental shape.

I've watched men on the geriatrics service of the mental hospital where I work. Many of them are admitted in wheel chairs, having not been encouraged to become physically active or even to walk on their own. I've noticed that when the vigorous program the treatment team starts with them gets them off their duffs and physically active again, many of the men actually become interested again in the opposite sex! Proof positive that you have it in you all the time to maintain adequate sex hormones.

TO TAKE OR NOT TO TAKE HORMONES

Almost every day I'm asked, "When do I start my hormone shots?" This, mostly from women. I tell them all the same thing: "You don't!" There are actually two conditions women experience at or near menopause that can be helped by taking hormones, and both are temporary. The hormones can be stopped when the symptoms disappear. These two conditions are:

1. Hot flashes.
2. Drying out of mucous membranes (as in the lining of the vaginal vault).

Hormones will rapidly correct either one of these distressing symptoms. The hormones given are estrogens much like the ones the ovary produces during the premenopausal period. They are always taken by mouth. They need *never* be taken by shot. In fact, the local application of hormone cream, in the case of vaginal drying out, is quite satisfactory.

Insofar as men are concerned, there are *no* indications for taking testosterone that I'm aware of. The sale and promotion of such hormones "to stimulate renewed sexual prowess" in men is about as effective as taking plain water. And much more expensive!

THE STORY OF BIRTH CONTROL HORMONES

The most talked about subject today among women is the taking of "the pill." And for good reason. It's one of the major medical breakthroughs of the century. The "pill" is a hormone that suppresses (stops) ovulation for as long as it's used. If there's no ovulation, there's no fertilization; hence, no pregnancy.

Like everything else in the world, "the pill" is not for everybody. And like virtually every other drug on the market today, including aspirin, if enough people take enough pills, somebody is going to have some unwanted side-effects from taking it. It's been demonstrated clearly enough, as far as I'm concerned, that the pill is a safe, effective birth control method if used properly. And what does "properly" mean, exactly? It means just as prescribed by your doctor. Furthermore, I believe that after a year or two of marriage, and taking the pill for birth control, a good thing to consider is the IUD as a reasonable substitute. The IUD (intra uterine device) is not a drug, hence, cannot cause drug side effects.

The following "myth table" will help clear up misunderstandings about "the pill."

> Myth: You will get serious blood clotting disorders on "the pill."
>
> Fact: You stand less chance of getting blood clot disorders from taking "the pill" than you would from having major surgery.

Myth: You turn into a "menopausal capon" on "the pill."

Fact: You don't turn into anything on "the pill." You may tend to collect some fluid in your tissues during the third week of the four weeks cycle, but this disappears when the pill is stopped during the fourth week.

Myth: "The pill" causes a prolonged delay in normal menopause.

Fact: Nonsense! No evidence from any study has shown this to be true.

Myth: Sometimes, the pill causes women to stop menstruating for the rest of their lives, long after "the pill" is stopped.

Fact: Sometimes "the pill" causes women to go without periods for sometimes weeks, or even months, but they invariably start again with time and patience.

Myth: "The pill" alters sex life.

Fact: If anything, it makes sex more interesting.

Myth: There are no serious drawbacks to "the pill."

Fact: Some women become unduly depressed while taking the pill. If this happens, the pill should be stopped. It's not known at this point whether the depression is wrapped in the woman's desires to become pregnant and she is frustrated in so doing, or whether it is physiological.

HORMONES THE ANSWER
TO PERPETUAL YOUTH?

This is a fair and good question. I think the answer is no. Hormones have been supplied to the aging in their normal physiological amounts in attempts to forestall the inevitable. All without success.

Actually, we're talking about two different questions entirely — that of keeping youthfully tuned organisms for all of our "three score and ten," and that of "living forever." I'm not certain at this point that the latter will ever become something to strive for, but it may be possible to materially prolong the seventy-odd years given most of us to sojourn on this earth, or other planets, in the future. I am convinced that whatever is discovered in future to prolong our lives will most certainly depend on the duality that I've spoken of many times in this book and elsewhere: in the smooth and efficient interlocking of a healthy body with a sound mind.

I think a much better approach to the problem at this stage of the human condition is found in the idea behind this book. Namely, that of keeping a youthful, vital, sound organism for as long as the good Lord allows us to remain on tap.

CHAPTER SUMMARY

1. Hormones are potent chemical regulators in your body. Their farflung actions would fill a separate book. In keeping youthful luster in your tissues, your hormones are an important adjunct.

2. Your master endocrine gland, the pituitary, is known to be under the influence of extremely potent neurohormones coming from special cells located in the emotion center of your brain. Another excellent reason for gaining mind control in keeping young.

3. The much-talked about difference in male and female hormones are really not that much different. The same set of rules apply to keeping youthful male hormones as in sustaining youthful female hormones.

4. "The pill" is a much maligned but important factor in keeping down the population in our country. It's beneficial effects far outweigh its potential hazards at this stage of our knowledge.

14

How to Use Vitamins
to Sustain Youthfulness

There are some things you should know about the subject of vitamins to complete your youth-building picture. These bits of information will help you in maintaining youthful tone.

The kinds of vitamins, what they do, where they're found — this knowledge is important. I want to talk about it in this section. The converse, or what vitamins won't do, is equally important for you to know. This will be covered as well.

There is a place in your body for the known vitamins. Each has its specific function in specific reactions vital to your metabolism, hence, in the maintenance of tissues. Obviously, a shortage of such a specific vitamin could intensify the aging of that particular tissue. I want you to understand what to do about insuring that you won't short yourself in vitamin content.

It is probably true that there are vitamins that haven't been recognized as yet — the ones we do know about weren't all discovered together, but through years of analysis and study. Perhaps one day we will identify a vitamin that our body needs, and manufactures for a time, that will materially prolong the efficient life of the single cell. I will point out in this section how research in this field is progressing.

VITAMINS, WHAT ARE THEY?

Vitamins are the great organic catalysts of your organism. A catalyst is any substance that alters or changes a chemical reaction, but remains generally unaltered itself. For instance, two chemicals are mixed together in a test tube. Immediately, an intense reaction occurs with the production of a lot of heat and bubbling, then it stops. Mix the same two chemicals together, but this time do so with a small piece of metal, say, platinum, in the test tube and the reaction goes ahead slowly, evenly, with the giving-off of a constant, even heat over a period of time. In such a reaction, the piece of platinum is the catalyst — it changes the way the two chemicals react with each other, but remains unaltered itself in the process.

Vitamins, then, change the way many life processes progress in your body, but themselves aren't involved much in the reactions. But they do wear out and have to be replaced.

In general, there are two kinds or types of vitamins. Water soluble and fat soluble. This means that the water soluble vitamins can be absorbed into your system just by being mixed with water. The fat soluble vitamins, on the other hand, must be dissolved into the oils and fats in your diet. This is why people who use a lot of mineral or olive oil may be short on vitamins — they don't get a chance to get absorbed. This will become important as we discuss the sources of vitamins further along in this section.

In general, also, vitamins are a group of seemingly completely unrelated substances. That is, they don't come from a similar family of chemicals or appear similar when their formulas are written out.

A few vitamins can be synthesized in your body. Most of the so-called B vitamins can be manufactured by the bacteria normally present in your intestinal tract. Most vitamins, however, must be taken in the food you eat as the body seems unable to make them. The reason for this curious fact isn't known.

WHAT VITAMINS DO

Vitamin A

This vitamin is one of the fat soluble ones. It is vital for growth and development in children. This is why it is given to babies. In adults, the vitamin is essential for preservation of good vision and healthy skin.

Vitamin B Complex

The B vitamins are several in number and grouped together for simplicity's sake. Riboflavin and thiamine, two common names seen on cereal boxes, and bread wrappers, and so on, are two of the most widely recognized B complex vitamins. They are essential in blood formation, skin and mucous membrane, health, nerve and muscle tissue function, and the manufacture of protein.

Vitamin C

Often called ascorbic acid, this vitamin is found in abundance in fresh fruits, especially citrus fruits. It is vital to the health of the "cellular cement" tissues — the connective tissue I've talked about that forms the elastic tissue in your skin and that forms the inside linings of your blood vessels.

Vitamin D

This vitamin, also a fat soluble vitamin like Vitamin A, plays the crucial role in control of your calcium cycle and in phosphorous metabolism. Children who don't get enough vitamin D have rickets. In adults, it plays an important part in the formation of the hormone manufactured by your parathyroid glands.

Vitamin E

The third and final fat soluble vitamin, vitamin E probably plays a basic role in the process of reproduction, though exactly how or what it does in this field hasn't been worked out as yet. Recently, it has been suggested that vitamin E is essential to the elimination of the "clinkers" that collect in cells as a result of their slowing down, thus it may prove to be an anti-aging vitamin.

Vitamin K

This vitamin is vital to the blood clotting mechanism in your system. It is often used routinely in newborn infants or in mothers just before delivery to prevent serious hemorrhage.

Not too long ago, there were vitamins L through X. These substances have since been found either not to be vitamins or else to be alterations of the main vitamins listed above.

This table will help you determine the sources of vitamins.

VITAMIN	*WHERE FOUND	CAUTIONS
A	Fish liver and liver oils. All vegetables, especially "orange" vegetables (carrots, squash, etc.).	At least one serving of "orange" vegetable daily. Do not use mineral or olive oil with such foods.
B	Very widespread — beef liver and meats, yeast, flour, wheat germ, cereals, etc. Intestinal bacteria manufacture.	Use in large quantities when on antibiotics.
C	Citrus fruits (oranges, grapefruit, lemons, limes, fruit juice).	Not stored in body. One or two servings of citrus fruit daily. Easily broken down by exposure to air, light and heat.
D	Fish liver and liver oils, pasteurized milk (milk that has been irradiated).	Oils and fats prevent absorption.
E	Green leafy vegetables, vegetable oils, cereals and nuts. Wheat Germ oil.	Oils and fats prevent absorbtion. Stored in body.

*See page 185 for a more detailed list.

There has been much written and suggested about what vitamins are supposed to do for you. Every so many years, it becomes the vogue to suggest to people that if a little vitamin therapy is good, then a lot of vitamins are all the better. This is *not* so.

With the exception of the fat soluble vitamins — A, D and E — when you take in a wad of vitamins that your body can't use almost immediately, your body simply excretes them through the stool or urine. The fat soluble vitamins are capable of being stored to a certain extent in your body for future use, but it is possible to overuse these vitamins — and when they're overused, they can make you quite ill!

Virtually every dread disease state — the rare disorders that are seen only once in a blue moon — have been treated with high doses of vitamins by perfectly competent research doctors and scientists. All results have been uniform. They didn't help at all! So there is no sense at all in overloading anybody with vitamins they don't need or can't use.

It's also a convenience to blame a host of ills, real and imaginary, on "low vitamins." If a person feels below par, he goes to the drug store and buys a bottle of vitamins from which he religiously takes two or three every day. I wish I could say this would work wonders, but it doesn't. Your body can handle the vitamin problem easily if you'll just follow the table on the preceding page and on the last page.

WHEN YOU NEED VITAMINS

There are times when extra vitamins will help. Taking them at the proper times will aid in keeping youthful healthy tissues.

Illness

It's safe to say that any illness you may have that keeps you off your feet for longer than a couple of days will cause a vitamin shortage in your system. This includes surgery if you can't get back on good dietary intake in a couple of days. For the usual illness that keeps you in bed at home, and off a good diet, almost any of the vitamin tablets or capsules will suffice. One, or at the most, two of these a day, is plenty. Remember, your body has stored vitamins A, D and E. If the vitamins you are taking don't have much, if any, of these vitamins in them, don't feel shortchanged — you probably don't need to take them.

During your recovery, plenty of fresh fruits and juices will add vitamin C to your system. Since this vitamin is vital to repair of diseased tissue and in the repair of wounds, it pays to take plenty of vitamin C.

If you need to, Brewers yeast tablets are an excellent source of the B complex vitamins. They're quite digestible and most inexpensive, a thousand tablets can be purchased for a dollar and a half or less. The usual daily dose is twelve tablets daily. They are a good regulator of the bowels as well.

Dieting

During prolonged dieting to get off excess pounds, you might short yourself on vitamins. It is well to insure against this while dieting by taking a good vitamin preparation containing A, D and E as well as the others, since your body stores these vitamins in its fatty tissue. But don't let this stop you from dieting. Your body can always find enough fat tissue to store these vitamins in when you've lost weight — it doesn't take very much fat tissue for such storage.

Antibiotics

When you're on antibiotics for any length of time (and there are some conditions that may require you to be) you need extra vitamins. The reason for this is that the antibiotics destroy the "good" bacteria in your system as well as the "bad" ones. The "good" bacteria in your intestinal tract are the ones that help absorb vitamins from the food you eat and help manufacture certain vitamins (like B complex, for instance). When these "good" bacteria are disabled, extra vitamins are indicated, especially ones with large amounts of vitamin B and C complex.

Other Reasons

These are rare, indeed. It used to be that many conditions besetting certain groups of humans in our world altered diets such that vitamins as well as almost all other essential food-stuffs were in serious depletion. For instance, men sailing on long voyages aboard ship often got pellagra or scurvy from lack of B and C vitamins respectively. The reason was primarily that they got no fruit aboard ship. Any situation you may be in where your regular diet is altered for prolonged periods of time will, of course, necessitate your taking vitamins. Unless you're planning prolonged trips to the bush country of Africa or such, I can't imagine these circumstances being encountered very often.

Recently, I read a newspaper story of a Nobel Prize winning scientist (a biochemist) who said he routinely takes about four to six *grams* of extra vitamin C every day because he thought that his studies had "led me to suspect that it might help me fight off disease and stay younger!" He said he took the extra vitamin C in the form of "four to six tablespoons of Ascorbic acid powder" every day.

Now, I can't say whether this scientist is doing the right thing or not. He *is* looking quite young at the age of about seventy years, but might be doing just as well had he not been using the extra vitamin C. I honestly don't know. I do know that neither this distinguished scientist nor anyone else, at our present stage of knowledge, can tell us why we should eat extra vitamins or, if so, in what quantity, or even what we might expect from them. Maybe this eminent scientist is doing the right thing. I think we should wait and see. I think we should concentrate on all the things we *know* revitalize and preserve youth — these, at least, are tried and true!

CHAPTER SUMMARY

1. Vitamins are essential for youth and health. Fortunately, they are found widely in good general diets unless you are avoiding certain foods routinely.

2. Some vitamins are soluble in fats and oils. Animal and mineral oils should not be used to excess or over prolonged periods of time because these oils may prevent the absorption of Vitamins A, D, and E.

3. There are certain types of stress that require extra vitamins. These include chronic illness, surgery with debilitation, antibiotics prescribed over long periods and other rare reasons. Any vitamin product will give adequate protection during these times of stress.

IMPORTANT FOOD SOURCES OF VITAMINS

Vitamin A	Fish liver oils	Butter
	Liver and kidney	Margarine
	Vegetables —	Fortified cream

IMPORTANT FOOD SOURCES OF VITAMINS

	green and yellow Fruits — yellow Tomatoes, tomato products Egg yolk	Cheese — from whole milk
Vitamin B Complex	Yeast Organ meats — liver and heart Meat and poultry Soybeans Oysters Potatoes Peas Eggs Mushrooms	Whole grain and enriched cereals Melons Milk Vegetable greens Wheat germ Beans Peanut butter
Vitamin C	Citrus fruits Melons Berries Tomatoes	Vegetables — especially raw peppers, broccoli, cauliflower, kale, brussel sprouts, turnip greens, and cabbage
Vitamin D	Fish liver oils Fat fish, liver	Fortified milk (pasteurized) Egg yolk
Vitamin E	Wheat germ Seed germ oils Vegetable greens Vegetable oils	Pod vegetables Cereal products Egg yolk Nuts
Vitamin K	Vegetable greens Cabbage Soybean oil	Tomatoes Cauliflower Vegetable oils

So, unless you are on a strict diet for some reason, it's very difficult to end up short of vitamins. If you *are* on a diet, and it needn't be forever, you can and should take extra vitamins for youthful nutrition, as I've already mentioned. Look at the labels on the vitamin bottles in the drugstore. It will tell you how much of the daily requirement of each vitamin you will get by taking the preparation. The most expensive is not necessarily the most vitamin-rich.

15

How to Restore Youthful
Go-Power Even Though
Diabetes Tries to Slow
You Down

Diabetes is a disease that interferes with blood sugar levels. In this section I'd like to take a look at what diabetes is, what it does to your system and how you can shed years from your body in spite of it. Most important, I'd like to show you how you can prevent diabetes. I'll point out why it's important to prevent it — why you'll be years ahead in preventing heart and blood vessel disease if you keep diabetes out of the picture.

If diabetes *has* started, I'd like to show you how to take care of it, and how you can continue good principles of youth-building in dealing with it. I'll cover the role of diet, insulin injections and pills.

It's important to know how to test your urine in controlling diabetes as well as about important tests done in a laboratory such as the glucose tolerance test. I'll talk about these tests.

WHAT IS DIABETES?

Diabetes is a failure of the endocrine system to burn sugar properly. Sugar collects in the blood stream in high amounts, and this *high level* of blood sugar starts a series of events that causes far-reaching problems with the entire metabolism.

The diabetic "trait" has long been recognized as hereditary. That is, the defect in diabetes can be transmitted from one generation to the next, depending on a number of factors. Sometimes, diabetes is seen in a generation of children where either mother or father has the disease. At other times, diabetes may be present in one or both grandparents, not present in any of their children, but crop up again in one or more of the grand-children. There are still other factors that don't depend on heredity.

At the outset, I think it's well to consider diabetes from three distinct angles. These are as follows:

1. *Juvenile diabetes.* This variety brings the worst possible features of the disease to the forefront. In juvenile diabetes, the symptoms start at an early age, sometimes as early as six years, usually in the teens. Since this period in life represents a phase of rapid growth when a youngster is changing metabolically at an enormous pace anyway, diabetes is difficult to recognize and control.
2. *Adult diabetes.* This form of the disease is the most common. It may hit suddenly, but it's generally slow in starting. Recognized early, adult diabetes can be quickly and efficiently controlled.
3. *Late-onset diabetes.* This form of diabetes comes on late in life, after the fifth decade or so. It is milder in nature and most likely to respond to conservative measures of control than the other two forms.

Juvenile Type: What Are It's Signs?

Jay, age nine, is an example of what I mean. Jay was brought to the office in a semi-comotose condition; that is, he was unconscious and responding weakly. His unconscious state had occurred suddenly at school during recess. Jay was a reasonably well and active boy who had lost a little weight, according to his mother's story later, but since his appetite had slackened, the weight loss seemed normal. Jay's urine test, done immediately in the office indicated large amounts of sugar and acid compounds, a situation demanding hospitalization and emergency measures.

Acid compounds in the urine, called ketones, means that the body has called on fat stores for the production of calories (energy) since the lack of insulin makes it impossible to burn carbohydrates (the source of sugar, remember) for energy. When fats are used for such energy burning, large amounts of acid are left over from this emergency use of food stores. The acid had made Jay lapse into a coma because his body couldn't neutralize it fast enough.

Jay recovered promptly, and has been taking insulin since this time. His diet and activity have been regulated well by his parents so that Jay's growth and development have proceeded normally. Jay happens to be a good athlete, and is able to enjoy sports to the fullest in spite of his diabetes. He is being encouraged to continue so that he'll delay an early aging process!

Adult Type

Vi was thirty-two, married five years and pregnant with her first child when she came to me. She was about five months along, had gained thirty pounds over the past three months and was miserable. She told me that she drank "quarts of water every day" and spent most of her time in the bathroom urinating. She was weak, tired quite easily and noted swelling of her feet and lower legs. She thought her pregnancy was causing all the symptoms. Unfortunately, diabetes was the culprit. It's unusual to have gained such weight so early in pregnancy. In fact, it's well that one's total weight gain doesn't exceed twenty pounds at the end of pregnancy.

Insulin was again necessary for Vi, as was a severe restriction of diet so she could get her weight in line, yet get enough nourishment for herself and her unborn child. Another drug to stimulate her kidneys to pump out the excess fluid was also necessary. Vi's baby was delivered somewhat past her due date, a normal situation with most diabetic mothers. Her baby was large and had a bit of trouble breathing at birth — also expected with diabetes. But the baby is well and thriving today, and Vi has been able to keep her diabetes under excellent control, a problem she found much easier after her baby was born. One of Vi's grandparents had diabetes of the late onset type. Neither of her parents had the disease. Although Vi could tolerate further pregnancies, she has been advised not to become pregnant again. She will add years to her comfortable life span if she has no further children.

Late Onset Type

Cora is sixty-nine years old and a grandmother of six. She had a rather difficult life when rearing her family of seven, but had enjoyed good health in spite of her family's hard times. She began to add weight when she reached fifty, and had slowly added more until she was forty-five pounds overweight. She, too, noticed increasing weakness, increased thirst and increased urine output, spells of nausea and vomiting without pain or cramps in her abdomen. A check showed mild diabetes.

Cora responded surprisingly well to weight loss and to one of the newer tablets designed to stimulate the production of insulin. All her symptoms disappeared, and she is well and active today. Cora has learned to live with her disease.

WHEN THE PANCREAS STOPS
PRODUCING INSULIN SUFFICIENTLY

In young Jay's case just described, and in all cases of juvenile diabetes, the pancreas gland just plain gives out. The pancreas, remember, is the endocrine gland that makes insulin. And insulin is necessary to metabolize sugar (to burn it as energy) inside each of the trillions of cells in your body.

This sudden giving out requires immediate corrective steps, and the first of these is giving insulin from another source. Unlike adult diabetes, the child's pancreas isn't capable of being stimulated to make even a little insulin. The fact that when the adult pancreas plays out, it doesn't *quit altogether,* is what makes it possible to use medicines taken by mouth to bring it under control. Such diabetic pills, as they're sometimes called, stimulate the "flagged-out" pancreas to perform more nearly up to snuff. With the child, there is no more reserve. Insulin must be supplied in all cases.

The pancreas gland contains several kinds of cells in its substance. At least one of these cell varieties does the insulin-making, and the insulin is emptied directly into your blood stream where it reaches virtually every cell in your body in a matter of seconds.

In an adult, when the pancreas begins to wear down, other changes also take place. There is, for example, a change in the way both carbohydrate and fat are handled in the body. Fat metabolism depends on the intactness of carbohydrates and sugar metabolism. Disturb one, and the rest are likewise disturbed. People with diabetes always have disturbances in fat deposition. In fact, abnormal fat acquisition — too much fat — can trip the switch that starts the diabetic process. In my experience, *no* fat person ever has truly normal carbohydrate metabolism. Furthermore, 90 percent of people who are too fat most of their lives will eventually develop the diabetic state if they live long enough. This is true regardless of whether or not they have diabetes in their family history. Fat is, indeed, anti-youth!

Ruby, a woman in her forties, was always overweight. When I first met her, she was about five feet five and weighed 220 pounds! When she developed diabetes, it came under good control with insulin after a hopeless few months at trying to get her to lose weight so she could get by with pills for her diabetes. She tried to cooperate with weight reduction; but in spite of rigid control of her calories, she continued to gain, and at a more rapid rate after starting insulin that before!

In the hospital, tests showed Ruby also had an extremely high blood fat level. It was also discovered that she had hardening of the arteries of a rather severe nature, a condition that wouldn't be expected for at least another twenty-five to thirty years! Finally, with control of her insulin to a fine point and with a special diet that severely restricted carbohydrates *and fats,* her blood levels of fat began to drop slowly down to normal. With this drop in fats, at least the hardening artery process was arrested!

Ruby illustrates why some people are unable to reduce, in fact may gain, in spite of careful effort on their part to lose weight. The idea of their fat metabolism also being altered isn't taken into proper account. And it's because of this altered fat metabolism that people with diabetes have a tendency to have coronary artery disease and strokes — their blood vessels suffer because this circulating fat gets deposited on the inside lining and causes plugs to form in their arteries. Do you begin to see why doctors always seem to be harping at people because of their excess weight?

REVERSING THE DIABETIC ORGAN AGING PROCESS

Kidneys

There are many thousands of diabetics in this country today who can thank their lucky stars their diabetes was discovered when it was. When diabetes first begins, there is an elevated level of sugar, as you now know, in the blood stream. Your kidneys have the task, remember, of filtering out everything in the fluid portion of your blood as it flows through them, sorting out the wastes and refiltering vital substances back into your blood again. The wastes, of course, pass into the urine where they are eliminated. When your blood sugar level goes beyond a certain point, sugar begins to "spill-out" in the urine. Kidneys aren't able to re-filter all of it back into your system. The presence of sugar in your urine is abnormal since no sugar is "spilled" if carbohydrates are being used by your cells in the normal way. The fact that some sugar is usually spilled serves to make testing the urine for sugar a useful screening test for diabetes.

Some kidneys have higher "thresholds" for spilling sugar than others. By this, I mean that patient A may spill sugar when his blood sugar level is, say, 175. Patient B may spill sugar when his blood sugar is 280. (The normal fasting blood sugar level is between seventy and one hundred mg. %.) In this case, patient B is said to have a high threshold for sugar, and patient A, a normal threshold.

The point is that urine testing for diabetes is not fool-proof. Sometimes, only a fasting blood sugar level or a *glucose tolerance test* will bring out the diagnosis of diabetes.

Kidneys may suffer through changes in their structure in long-standing diabetes. These changes have nothing to do with the sugar that spills during the early stages of diabetes. It does have to do with hardening of the tiny artery capillaries in the filter system — and the disease that's produced is similar to what I've already talked about in relation to arteries elsewhere in the body — the arteries harden and fail to carry blood properly. When this occurs in the kidneys, the filter system fails to work properly for the wastes the kidney must constantly get rid of. These wastes pile up in the system and cause much difficulty. Fortunately, good control of diabetes when it first pops up, coupled with careful attention to principles of blood sugar control afterward, can prevent such "aging" changes in your kidneys.

Eyes

Yet another complication of diabetes is cataracts. Cataracts are opaque blobs that appear in the lens of the eyes. They're fairly common in people of advanced age, but occur much

earlier in diabetes. They're caused by faulty fat and carbohydrate metabolism. These poorly broken down substances are
deposited in the lens of the eye for as yet unknown reasons.
If you happen to have diabetes and if you haven't taken good
care of your youth controls, cataracts may result.

A man named Rod recently presented himself in the emergency room at a hospital having suddenly gone blind in the
right eye. He was thirty-eight years old, and considered himself in good health. He was a large, flabby person, about 55
pounds overweight for his height and frame. He obviously
didn't get much exercise, since just walking from his car to the
hospital emergency area caused him to huff and puff like a
threshing machine. Rod, of course, was in a panic. He said he
noted some pain in the back of his eye earlier at work, then
all vision vanished on the right side.

On looking inside his eye with the gadget used to examine
the retina, it was clear what had happened. He'd had a sudden
occlusion (plugging-up) of the small opthalmic blood vessel,
the one that comes directly into the eye with the large nerve
that enables you to see. Several things can cause this to happen,
but in Rod's case, it was diabetes. When his disease came under
control and anticoagulant drugs given, the artery partially un-
plugged, enabling Rod to see fairly well out of this eye again.
His vision will never be quite the same, but he's lucky that he
has any sight left.

The arteries do age prematurely with diabetes, and everything I've discussed regarding the blood vessels and heart *apply
all the more* with diabetes. There's only one way to forestall
diabetic agony: *prevent diabetes in the first place by adhering
to the principles of youth-building.* Rod didn't, and he's paying
for it now.

Do diabetics have more strokes than others because of this
aging artery vulnerability? Yes, they do, *but this too can be
prevented by following the principles of youth control* and if
diabetes has already started, these principles are *all the more
important!*

Nervous System

Even your nervous system is vulnerable in the diabetic state.
Because the sheath that surrounds nerves in the body depend

on a constant supply of carbohydrate to keep the delicate fibers inside them "insulated" so they work properly, anything that disrupts carbohydrate turnover in the body will eventually affect nerves.

I recently saw a man who was a diabetic and an alcoholic, and who had been unable to control his drinking problem. He took insulin for his diabetes, but frequently went on long binges where his insulin, his diet and his physical tone went to pot. Finally, he came out from an alcoholic stupor one day unable to make his legs work properly. At first, it was thought that he had some lingering toxic effects from the alcohol, but the problem progressed until his right lower and left upper leg muscles were paralyzed. He had pain in both legs as well, and occasionally had to be given narcotics to stop it. He had destruction of some of the large nerves to his legs as a result of prolonged poor control of his diabetes. This condition is called diabetic neuropathy. The nerves involved can be most anywhere in the body, and their destruction is largely permanent once it occurs — one more reason for taking better care of yourself *before* diabetes starts, or if started, an undeniable argument in favor of following good youth retaining principles.

HOW DIABETES IS TREATED

Insulin

The drug the pancreas normally makes in your body is insulin. It follows that a shortage might be helped by supplying what is missing. Insulin used to be derived from cow and hog pancreas. It has now been made synthetically. Insulin used to come out in one form. Now it comes in several. The most widely used type is the so-called NPH type, so designated to indicate that it starts to work and has its peak activity after injection in the middle range of all the various insulins. Regular insulin, for example, goes to work in minutes after it's injected. It's peak is within a couple of hours, then it rapidly disappears from the system. This is why people with diabetes used to have to take their insulin several times a day.

Yet another insulin is quite delayed in its action, but stays in the system for several hours once it starts to act. NPH is in the middle of these two ranges. NPH goes to work an hour or two after it's injection and it has its peak activity shortly after noon, if it's taken in the morning on arising. It then tapers off slowly. NPH is versatile because usually, a diabetic person can do with only one injection a day in the morning. Sometimes, however, another dose is necessary, usually regular insulin, late in the afternoon or in the evening.

Whatever the schedule, the present day insulins are safe, effective and pure.

Pills

In the past ten years, at least four different drugs have been developed for the oral treatment of diabetes. Some have as their action the stimulation of the insulin-producing cells in your pancreas. The lazy cells are prodded to release insulin. Others don't have any effect at all on the pancreas, but appear to be "insulin substitute" agents whose precise actions aren't well understood at the present time. At any rate, these drugs have been of inestimable help in the management of diabetes.

Their chief help has been with the late-onset type of diabetes, and in non-severe types. Many of our oldsters with diabetes have been spared the chore of having to take insulin injections by using such drugs. They have little or no place in the treatment of juvenile diabetes because the pancreas in the juvenile is completely exhausted. Insulin is the only drug for diabetes in the youngster.

Diet

Here we are again. Right back to diet, the anchor chain in the treatment of diabetes. Whatever I've said to this point about diet in the prevention of disease and in maintaining youth, you may be certain that it applies fifty-fold when diabetes has entered the picture. Exactly the same principles apply. If you have diabetes, for example, and are too heavy — *you must reduce!* If you have diabetes and are underweight, *you must get your weight up!*

The foods in the diabetic diet aren't generally measured with a scale like they used to be. It's been shown that people need varying amounts of energy calories according to what their activities are during a given time. This means everybody's energy requirement varies from week to week, even day to day. It's also known how much a person of a given weight needs in the way of protein, carbohydrate and fat to have efficient metabolism and to thrive. It's on this basis that diabetic diets today are calculated with allowances for more or less physical activity.

It's common sense that if you have diabetes, and are extra active, you will need during that day, that week or whatever, both extra energy and extra insulin to burn this energy.

DIABETIC URINE TESTS

I've discussed the role of the kidney in diabetes — that when the level of sugar rises to a particular height in the blood stream, sugar leaks into the urine. It's this event that forms the basis for following the control of diabetes at home once the disease has come under medical care and treatment. It works this way:

1. In the hospital laboratory, your blood levels of sugar have been measured.
2. At the same time this measurement was going on (the blood sugar tolerance test) a urine sample was also tested as each blood test was done. This urine testing lets your doctor know at what blood level sugar "spilled over" in your urine. Say, for example, that at a blood level of 250 your urine showed a two or three plus reaction on the strip of test tape used to test urine sugar.
3. You now have the means to come very close to knowing where your blood sugar level is by testing urine at home, using this same tape that you simply dunk into a small sample of your urine. You want to keep your urine test between a trace to one plus on the color scale on the side of the test tape container and a *negative* test for acid. This way, your blood sugar is just a bit high — the *safest* place for it to be. To get it any lower may mean you'll have an insulin reaction from time to time. It's always best to keep a little sugar in the urine. You'll avoid insulin reactions and if for any reason (like an infection, for example) you need to boost your insulin dose, you'll be on the safe side in so doing.

The test tape comes in strips just long enough for one test. You simply place the end of the tape into a voided specimen of urine and compare the color change that takes place on the strip of tape with a standard color chart printed on the container. This chart will tell you how much sugar there is in your urine at this time.

When your diabetes is well-regulated, you won't need to test your urine every day, but you'll learn to test it when you don't feel just right or during certain other periods listed as follows:

1. During an infection. Sore throats, the "flu," a boil, sinusitis, diarrhea or bronchitis would be examples of common infections you might encounter. You will usually need *more* insulin or pills.
2. Increased physical activity. During vacations, week-end golf or hiking activities, adding exercise routines at home or having a baby are examples of increased activity you might encounter. If you take in more food, you'll need more insulin.
3. Surgery. Recuperation from any surgery speeds up metabolism. This requires more energy and this means more insulin if you have diabetes.
4. Unusual mental stress such as a death in the family, a shock, a mental illness or a chronic problem in the family that "takes it out of you" psychologically.

Remember, when such stress periods come to an end, your insulin requirements may well return to previous "standard levels" again — another reason for keeping just a little sugar showing in your urine. If a trace of sugar suddenly disappears, you suspect that your insulin dose or pill dose is too high and you can cut the dose down accordingly, and take in more carbohydrates.

YOUTHFUL VIGOROUS LIFE
IN SPITE OF DIABETES

Regardless of the troubles diabetes can cause, you can live a youthful and vigorous life with it. Remember these points:

Juvenile

1. Suspect diabetes in any child who isn't growing or developing properly; who drinks and urinates excessively; who
   has "behavior" problems or where one or both parents
   have the disease, or one of the grandparents has the
   disease.
2. After the age of seven years, any child can learn to give
   his own insulin injection — show patience, be firm and
   understanding and help him learn to check his urine
   with tape strips routinely.
3. Insulin requirements, diet and activity change rapidly
   in childhood. Be alert for such changes and adjust routines
   accordingly. Let him grow up in the same way you would
   if he didn't have the disease. Build the insulin and diet
   around what he does, *not* what he does around insulin and
   diet restrictions.
4. Teach him proper youth control principles.

Adult Late Onset

1. Suspect diabetes if there is excess thirst or urinating; a
   rash of infections anywhere, especially on the skin;
   prolonged excessive weight or sudden loss of weight;
   vision disturbances and excessive fatigue without physical
   cause for it.
2. Whether using oral drugs or insulin for diabetes, study
   the youth principles outlined in this book and adhere
   to them strictly from now on.
3. Test your urine at home with tape strips at intervals all
   the time, and more frequently during the stressful periods
   of physical and mental turmoil. Adjust insulin or pills
   accordingly. When in doubt, consult your doctor.
4. Remember that *exercise* always makes *diabetes more
   easily controlled* — at first, when you begin to exercise,
   your insulin requirements may rise somewhat, but later,
   you may be able to *reduce* your insulin and pill requirements.
5. Since NPH insulin has its peak just after noon if taken in
   the mornings, it's best to divide meals as follows: one-
   fifth breakfast; two-fifths lunch and two-fifths supper.

Add a mid-morning and mid-afternoon snack if you have any giddiness or shakiness.

Late Onset

1. This is the mildest form of diabetes, and the most likely to respond to oral drugs. Suspect diabetes of this type if you are past fifty-five years old and notice excess thirst and urinating; prolonged overweightness or sudden loss of weight; excessive fatigue for no physical reason; leg ulcers that don't heal well and eye disturbances of any kind.
2. Excessive physical and mental stresses may increase your need for control beyond oral drugs. Keep some *regular insulin* around in case you need to use it. Consult your doctor about how much to use and under what circumstances.
3. It's possible to take too much oral drug for diabetes just as it's possible to over-use insulin. Urine testing and attention to the signs of insulin reaction states will prevent this from happening.
4. You can and *should be physically active with diabetes.* Adjust your medicine or insulin according to what you're doing physically.

If you're following good youth principles, diabetes will be easy to handle. You have an excellent opportunity to practice preventive medicine with your youngsters if you're a diabetic. Have their urine checked frequently, teach them youth control and as they grow older, encourage them to follow the same procedures with your grandchildren!

CHAPTER SUMMARY

1. Diabetes is preventable in a large percentage of cases. Especially the adult type. The basic ground rules for preventions are the very ones already laid out for staying youthful: Diet, exercise and mind control. These rules should be followed even more rigorously if diabetes should appear.

2. The three types of diabetes are basically the same but appear in quite a different manner. Sudden, explosive and erratic in the young; slower more chronic and more steady of control in adults; slow, with secondary effects prominent in the late onset variety.

3. The blood vessels and heart, the nerves, the kidneys and eyes are affected in addition to the basic wearing out of the pancreas in diabetes. The better control of the disease, the less likely these complications are to appear. This means focus your attention on youth principles.

4. Building up insulin and diet (calories or energy) around your activity means a happier, healthier and more efficiently controlled diabetes. Don't let the disease run your life, let your youthful life principles control the disease.

5. The tape strip urine test is your best protection against shifts in your diabetes pattern. Test it often, test it regularly and test it carefully. The appearance of acid in your urine is much more significant than an occasional two or three pluses on the sugar scale. Both tests are usually on the tape strip. Get help from your doctor and take extra insulin if acid shows up.

16

Helpful Aids for Your Youth-Building Program

Dieting

When you're considering a diet, there are some things that will help guide you through the maze of details and misinformation and around all the jazzy and exotic diets that seem to enjoy cycles of popularity. The first thing to be considered by you in dieting is which foods are good and which bad? In Chapter Two, I discussed with you the question of carbohydrates, proteins and fat. The following table will help you become familiar with the foods you commonly eat.

TABLE OF FOOD CATEGORIES

Carbohydrate	Protein	Fat
Bread	Cereal	Meat fat
Candy	Cheese	Cream
Fruit	Egg	Butter
Margarine	Fish	Buttermilk
Potato	Flour	Cooking and
Plain milk	Meat	Salad oils
Pastries	Pod vegetable	Lard
Spaghetti and	(peas, corn, etc.)	Nuts
macaroni	Powder drinks	Chocolate
Soft drinks	Poultry	
Sugar	Yogurt, drained	
	cottage cheese	
	Skim and powdered	
	milk	

When you're trying to reduce, you need protein more than carbohydrate and carbohydrate more than fat. A good idea is to eliminate fats altogether for awhile, then, when your weight is down and you are getting back in physical tone, resume some fats again.

There are a few foodstuffs that can be considered calorie-free for practical purposes. These are:

1. All non-pod vegetables (carrots, lettuce, celery, etc.)
2. Crackers — plain and graham
3. Bouillon
4. Tea

I'm not saying that meals can or should be made up of these few foods. They will, however, help pull you through the periods where you feel starved and have uncomfortable hunger pangs. Between meals, eat two or three carrots. They won't upset your weight reduction plans, and they happen to be rich in vitamin A. They are also filling — they add "bulk" for your stomach walls to grind against, thereby relieving the hungry feeling you have. At bedtime, have a snack of some bouillon and crackers. Again, they relieve that empty feeling. Tea can be taken at mid-day for a "pick-me-up" snack along with some crackers.

There are a few vegetables that for some people are hard to digest. They are nourishing in that they contain good supplies of vitamins and minerals, and none of them will upset your weight losing plans, but if they seem to bother you, stay away from them. If they don't cause indigestion, then they, too, can be taken in most any amount without significantly adding calories. The list follows:

1.	Beans	7.	Onions
2.	Broccoli	8.	Peppers
3.	Brussel sprouts	9.	Radishes
4.	Cabbage	10.	Sauerkraut
5.	Cauliflower	11.	Turnips
6.	Cucumbers	12.	Parsnips

Under heavy fire these days from the Food and Drug Administration are the artificial sweeteners — especially cyclamates. I believe that the sweeteners used by diabetics for years, saccharin in either tablet or liquid form, remain safe and are a good way to restore the sweet taste to food and drink in place of using table sugar which is anti-weight-reducing.

LOW CHOLESTEROL DIET

I've discussed the role of cholesterol in producing disease and sludging of the inside lining of blood vessels in this book. Your coronary arteries and those in your head are vulnerable to being sludged when too much cholesterol is taken in your diet. Even if coronary disease or a stroke have already occurred it isn't too late to modify your diet so that at least there won't be progression of artery disease. If neither have entered the picture, you may prolong youth immeasurably by studying and following information regarding cholesterol:

FOOD GROUP	FOODS ALLOWED	FOODS TO AVOID
Beverages	Coffee, tea, coffee substitutes, carbonated beverages, skim milk, buttermilk made from skim milk	Whole milk, cream, Chocolate flavored beverages
Breads	Enriched white, whole wheat, rye, raisin, soda and graham crackers	Breads made with eggs, fats and oils
Cereals	Any with enriched or whole grain	Cereals containing chocolate
Cheese	Dry cottage cheese only	All others
Desserts	Cornstarch, bread rice, tapioca, junket, angel food cake, gelatin, sherbet, fruit ice, fruit whips, meringue, pastries, unsaturated fat pastries	All others

FOOD GROUP	FOODS ALLOWED	FOODS TO AVOID
Eggs	Egg white only	Egg yolk
Fats	Corn oil, margarine, soybeans and soy-bean oil, safflower oil, peanut oil, vegetable fat based toppings and cream substitutes, salad dressings made with any foregoing unsaturated fats	Butter, ordinary margarine, mayonnaise salad dressing, shortening, lard, suet
Fruit	All fruits and fruit juices	None
Meat, Fish, and Poultry	4-5 ounces meat/day: pork, ham, Canadian bacon, broiled, boiled or roast beef, lamb and veal, with no fat left on portions, chicken, turkey, most fish if packed in allowed oils (see above)	Bacon, brains, liver, sweet breads, heart, oysters, lobster, crab, shrimp. Fried meats, fish, or poultry unless fried in allowed fats (see above)
Seasonings	Salt, pepper, spices, herbs and extracts	None
Potato or substitute	White potato, sweet potato, yams, macaroni, noodles, spaghetti, rice, all with none but allowed oils	None
Soup	Meat broth without fat, bouillon, milk soups made with skim milk	Cream soups made with whole milk
Sweets	Sugar, jelly, jams, marmalade, honey,	Candy made with cream, chocolate

FOOD GROUP	FOODS ALLOWED	FOODS TO AVOID
	syrup, molasses, hard candy, gelatin candies, (gum drops, orange slices, and marshmallows).	or fat
Vegetables	Frozen, canned or fresh	None
Miscellaneous	Chili sauce, catsup, pickles, vinegar, cocoa, olives, nuts, baking chocolate, non-hydrogenated peanut butter	Gravy, milk chocolate, hydrogenated peanut butter

If you are both dieting for weight, and wish to be taking low cholesterol, the two diets can be made compatible by simply going through the above list and throwing out most of the fats and carbohydrates for your meals and substituting the allowable proteins until your weight is in line. Then, you may add some of the other allowable low cholesterol items to your diet.

THE LOW RESIDUE DIET

I talked about how to keep your gastro-intestinal system young earlier in this book, and mentioned that a low residue diet is quite helpful if you may be afflicted with temporary colitis, diverticulitis or other irritating gut inflammations. The diet is also useful following any surgery of the lower intestinal tract. The reason the diet is useful is that it keeps you away from a lot of food that leaves much bulk and irritating substances in your bowel to be later eliminated as large bulky stools. The diet that follows leaves a minimum of such residue for your bowel to cope with while you are restoring its youth.

FOOD GROUP	FOODS ALLOWED	FOODS TO AVOID
Beverages	Coffee, tea, sanka, carbonated beverages, cocoa, milk — one pint	Milk in excess of one pint a day.

FOOD GROUP	FOODS ALLOWED	FOODS TO AVOID
	daily, including that used in cooking.	
Breads	Toasted white bread, melba toast, soda crackers.	Coarse grain breads, hot breads, whole wheat bread, graham crackers.
Cereals	Cream of wheat, cream of rice, Malt-o-Meal, corn flakes, rice crispies, puffed rice, most refined cooked or dry cereals.	Ralston, Roman Meal, Wheatena, Wheaties, All Bran, Bran Buds, all other whole grain cooked or dry cereals.
Cheese	American and Swiss cheese used in cooking only. Cottage cheese, cream cheese.	All strongly flavored cheeses.
Desserts	Plain puddings, ice cream, sherbets, (these from milk allowance) gelatin, white, yellow and sponge cakes; sugar, vanilla and arrow-root cookies.	Pastries and desserts with nuts, coconut, raisins, seeds, and berries.
Eggs	All except fried.	Fried.
Fats	Butter, margarine, cream, white sauce, mayonnaise, bacon, plain gravy or milk gravy from milk allowance.	Nuts, coconut.
Fruits	Canned or soft cooked fruit cock-tail, peaches, pears, apples, peeled	All other fruits. No berries

FOOD GROUP	FOODS ALLOWED	FOODS TO AVOID
	apricots, bing cherries, royal anne cherries, pineapple, fruit juices may be used. Baked apples without skins, ripe banana, sectioned orange and grape-fruit.	
Meat, Fish or Poultry	Tender ground beef, lamb, veal, poultry, glandular meats, lean roast pork or ham, fish. All to be roasted, broiled or baked.	Highly seasoned meats, such as frankfurters, salami, bologna, all pickled meat, cured & spiced meat. Clams, oysters and sausage.
Potato and Substitute	White potato, rice, macaroni, noodles, and spaghetti.	Fried potatoes, potato skins, potato chips, sweet potato.
Soups	Broth, strained cream soups made from milk allow-ance, vegetable soup if made with allowed vegetables.	Commercial vegeta-ble soup, onions, and other highly seasoned soups.
Vegetables	Cooked asparagus tips, green or wax beans, beets, carrots, canned or pureed peas, pureed corn, chopped spinach, summer or mashed squash, tomato juice.	All raw vegetables. lettuce, celery, tomatoes, peppers, and onion.
Sweets	Moderate amounts of sugar, clear jellies, honey, syrup, marshmallows, hard	All others.

FOOD GROUP	FOODS ALLOWED	FOODS TO AVOID
	candy, gumdrops, milk chocolate, plain creams, (if diarrhea is present, all sweets to be eliminated).	
Miscellaneous	Salt, smooth peanut butter, paprika, parsley, vinegar, vanilla, cinnamon and mint.	Popcorn, pickles, spices, all seed-containing jams, pepper, mustard, catsup, sesame, poppy & caraway seeds.

ACNE

In treating and improving acne, as I discussed earlier in this book, the key is the elimination of fatty, greasy and oily foods that only make your somewhat overly oily skin more so. The following foods should be *eliminated completely* for good control of acne:

1. All fried foods. No exceptions.
2. All cola drinks. No exceptions.
3. Nuts, coconut, chocolate of all kinds.
4. Pastries, cheeses, pickled and cured meats.
5. All salad, cooking and other oils, butter and lard.

IDEAL WEIGHT FOR HEIGHT TABLES

MEN

Weight in pounds according to frame in indoor clothes.
Height (with shoes on — one inch heels)

Feet	Inches	Small Frame	Medium Frame	Large Frame
5	2	112-120	118-130	126-141
5	3	115-123	121-133	129-144
5	4	118-126	124-136	132-148
5	5	121-129	127-139	135-152

MEN

Feet	Inches	Small Frame	Medium Frame	Large Frame
5	6	124-133	130-143	138-156
5	7	128-137	134-147	142-161
5	8	132-141	138-152	147-166
5	9	136-145	142-156	151-170
5	10	140-150	146-160	155-174
5	11	144-154	150-165	159-179
6	0	148-158	154-170	160-184
6	1	152-162	158-175	168-189
6	2	156-167	162-180	173-194
6	3	160-171	167-185	178-199
6	4	164-175	172-190	182-204

WOMEN

Weight in pounds according to frame (In indoor clothing). Height (with shoes on — 2 inch heels)

Feet	Inches	Small Frame	Medium Frame	Large Frame
4	10	92-98	96-107	104-119
4	11	94-101	98-110	106-122
5	0	96-104	101-113	109-125
5	1	99-107	104-116	112-128
5	2	102-110	107-119	115-131
5	3	105-113	110-122	118-134
5	4	108-116	113-126	121-138
5	5	111-119	116-130	125-142
5	6	114-123	123-135	129-146
5	7	118-127	124-139	133-150
5	8	122-131	128-143	137-154
5	9	126-135	132-147	141-158
5	10	130-140	136-151	145-163
5	11	134-144	140-155	149-168
6	0	138-148	144-159	153-173

For girls between eighteen and twenty-five, subtract one pound for each year under twenty-five from weights given in tables.

Remember that Life Insurance Companies, whose job it is to *know, not guess* about life expectancy, have irrefutable

statistics that clearly show you will be healthier and live longer
— hence, stay younger — if you keep your weight close to the
lower figure given for the various height-frame categories.

Exercising

Remember that I emphasized in an earlier chapter that dieting and exercising (physical conditioning, toning, etc.) *cannot
and should never be considered separately.* Never think of one
without automatically thinking of the other. You'll remain
younger and healthier for the effort!

The key to taking the drudgery out of physical conditioning
is in developing new and different approaches to exercises.
Approaches that you, yourself, can make up if you just give a
little thought to it.

ISOMETRICS

For instance, you know that isometrics involve pitting one
group of muscles against its opposite group. There are isometrics
for every muscle group in your body. Your face for instance, can
be put through a short but extremely effective isometric routine
by starting with your chin muscles: flex your neck as far down on
your chest as you can get it. Now pull the muscle beneath your
chin — the one that has all these *extra* chins on it — as tightly
as you can, "smiling" with your mouth at the same time. Now
slowly draw up your chin until it points to the ceiling — as far
as your neck will bend back, in other words. Keep your under-
the-chin muscle stretched as tightly as you can all this while.
Now thrust out your lower jaw, keeping your chin stretched
tightly. Repeat this several times a night to get rid of that
double chin.

The rest of your face muscles are easy: just grimace as much
as you can — over and over again — smile as widely as your
mouth will go; pucker your lips as much as they'll pucker;
yawn widely and thrust your lower jaw from side to side; suck
in your cheeks until your mouth looks like a fish, then blow
your cheeks out using your hand to keep the air inside your
mouth.

Squint your eyes as tightly as you can — until you see
"stars." Wrinkle up your forehead muscles. You'll be surprised

at the youth you can restore to your face just by doing this simple routine every night!

You can put virtually any other muscle of your body through isometrics by making the particular muscle work against the opposite group. For instance, by gripping your clenched right fist with your left hand rotate your forearm palm down, then palm up. You put the main forearm muscle through an isometric. Now rotate it back again. Now do it reversing grips. See? You've mastered isometrics. The same applies to all your muscles. Be novel. Use your imagination. You can invent your own variations on the theme!

CALISTHENICS

Calisthenics are the more vigorous of exercises — sit-ups, scissor kicks and the like. When you want a real work-out, or when you want to start adding a little toughening up to your routine, start using calisthenics more. Do more of them at a time and different ones. For instance: when you've done well at doing sit-ups (remember, hands clasped behind neck during these, and no bending the knees!) start scissor kicks. These in the flat position on the floor, hands behind neck, legs about eighteen inches off the ground, and straight! Now swing them widely to the sides (until your groins pull) then back to the middle, crossing them over one another, left over right on the first swing, then right over left on the second. Keep knees straight at all times and no touching the floor with your heels!

Then when you can do these with ease, do the scissor clamps! These are doing sit-ups as described before, while, at the same time, doing the scissor kicks described above. When you can do thirty or forty of these, I guarantee you will have no further potbelly troubles!

Another good variation to use is the "track-starter." This is done by assuming the position you would if you were about to run the 440 in a track meet — that is, you squat down, one leg forward, the other backward, feet bent to "push-off," hands and arms supporting your weight in front. Now bring the leg that's back to the front, and the one that's in front, to the back — two of these front-back changes is one cycle. Do forty or fifty of these as you gather stamina and wind over a period of time. Your legs will grow stronger and you'll get some of that wind back!

Yet another variation is "jogging-in-place." You don't have to go outdoors for this one, just run, only hold your stationary position — move forward or backward as far as the room's dimensions or furniture will allow, yet keep the legs "running" all the while. As a further variation, you can squat down about every eight or ten "runs," then back up quickly to resume the running. Tremendous for the legs!

WEIGHTS

The rule of thumb for using weights is *caution* — caution with the weight you put on the bar itself and caution about doing too much too soon. If you take it easy with weights, they can be a helpful addition to your routines. You should never start out with more than twenty or thirty pounds of weights, balanced evenly on the bar. The trick to weights, as you will soon learn by experience, is balance — not brute strength. Remember, you're not trying to beat the world's record in amount of weights you can pick up and hoist in the air — you're trying to develop strength — gradually and in tune with your present state of conditioning. Don't overdo!

"Curling" with weights is done by grasping the bar close to the weights on either end, both in the palms up and the palms down positions, flexing the weights up and down, using your forearms to do the lifting. A variation on this is to let the weights hang down across your back side instead of your front. This way, the lifting is done with your shoulder and neck muscles as well as with your forearms.

Remember, you can approach your weight routines from any position — you don't simply have to just stand there and face the wall every time. You can squat down and put a different set of muscles into play by lifting the weights. You can lay down on the floor and thrust the weights up from their resting position across your chest (the bench press). You can kneel at the side of the weight as it rests on the floor and use one arm, then the other to lift it from its position.

And you can use the smaller weights (five to ten pounds) either singly or one in each hand to do circular motions at arms length, above your head, from the waist, etc. Learn to improvise — use as many sets of muscles as you can think of.

Extra Sensory Perception

In the fourth chapter, I discussed briefly the field of ESP (extra sensory perception). No doubt you've come across several ways while reading the rest of the book that mind control could help you immensely. Remember that your mind is the most potent tool you have in youth building. With and through your mind, you control all the keystones that go into making you look, feel and stay younger. Master your mind control. If you do, there are no limits out of reach!

In my opinion, ESP, a part of the mind, is one of the most fascinating and interesting of all the mysterious recesses of mind. There are many who put down the idea of ESP today — claim it's just a hoax, quite unworthy of time and energy. Yet I believe the last ten years has seen a slight softening of such rigid positions among scientists. Before he died, Albert Einstein even remarked that his theory of relativity was somehow connected with the business of ESP. I hope that the next ten years will see this subject get its long overdue intensive and imaginative research.

Meanwhile, there are ways you can strengthen your own ESP, based on the premise that ESP resides as part of all human minds (probably animal as well) awaiting only its development by all individuals.

AUTOSUGGESTION

You can use this portion of ESP as a means to help youth-building in a number of ways; for example, to start your physical conditioning routines. You need to get up a little earlier in the mornings to allow a bit of time for your before-breakfast toning. You need twenty or thirty minutes extra. So give yourself the suggestion to awaken thirty minutes earlier by your watch or bedroom clock. Give this suggestion repeatedly just as you are ready to doze off the night before (the optimum time for all such suggestions). Soon you will master the "mental alarm" that not only awakens you at definite and specific times, but also reminds you of chores, things to do, people to talk to, etc. during the day. Try it. Repeat it night after night. Don't give up until you've mastered it. You will, if you keep trying!

Another way to help your toning routines with autosuggestion is by concentrating very hard and very deeply before you start — concentrate on willing your muscles to do that extra two or three sit-ups, even though last time you tried them, you felt absolutely powerless to do even one more. You'll be surprised that you will, indeed, be able to get in more of the toners!

In concentrating, recall that you must put everything else out of your conscious mind for that short span of time — let nothing interfere with your repeated mental phrases to do or feel whatever it is you desire to do. Then, put the thought completely out of your conscious. Don't think about it again. Your subconscious will then take over and do your bidding!

Maybe at night, you "just don't have the vitality to do your toners." You can overcome this "no bazazz" business with about five minutes of autosuggestion. Just relax completely. Quietly, in a semi-darkened room, let yourself relax completely by concentrating on every part of your body to loosen up — go limp. When you've reached the stage of "twilight" (just before actual sleep comes), concentrate on vitality — "I will have strength, energy and the will to do the exercises" and repeat this over and over. At the end of five minutes or so, put the entire matter out of conscious mind. You'll be pleasantly surprised that within the next twenty or thirty minutes, a surge of robust electricity will pulsate through your body, and you'll actually want to exercise! You'll crave it, and feel better than you felt all day after you're through.

You can harness mind control in dieting to reduce weight. Simply repeat the phrase, "My appetite will be less. I won't crave food tomorrow." Repeat this, especially through those crucial first six weeks of dieting until your organism begins to adjust to the lessened food intake. You won't need pills. You won't need any crutches to get you eating less calories. Why? Because you've utilized your own resources — your mind — to do this job for you!

And it's only through an extension of this principle that you begin to use your mind to solve vexing problems, to get answers that won't come, to alter your attitudes toward others and to change the things about your personality that you know are aging your organism — worries, phantasies, nervousness and the like.

Use your ingenuity to the utmost in this field. The world is at your fingertips for your effort and you will once again be the vital, dynamic, youthful self you once were!

Index